Identifying And Controlling Pulmonary Toxicants

BACKGROUND PAPER

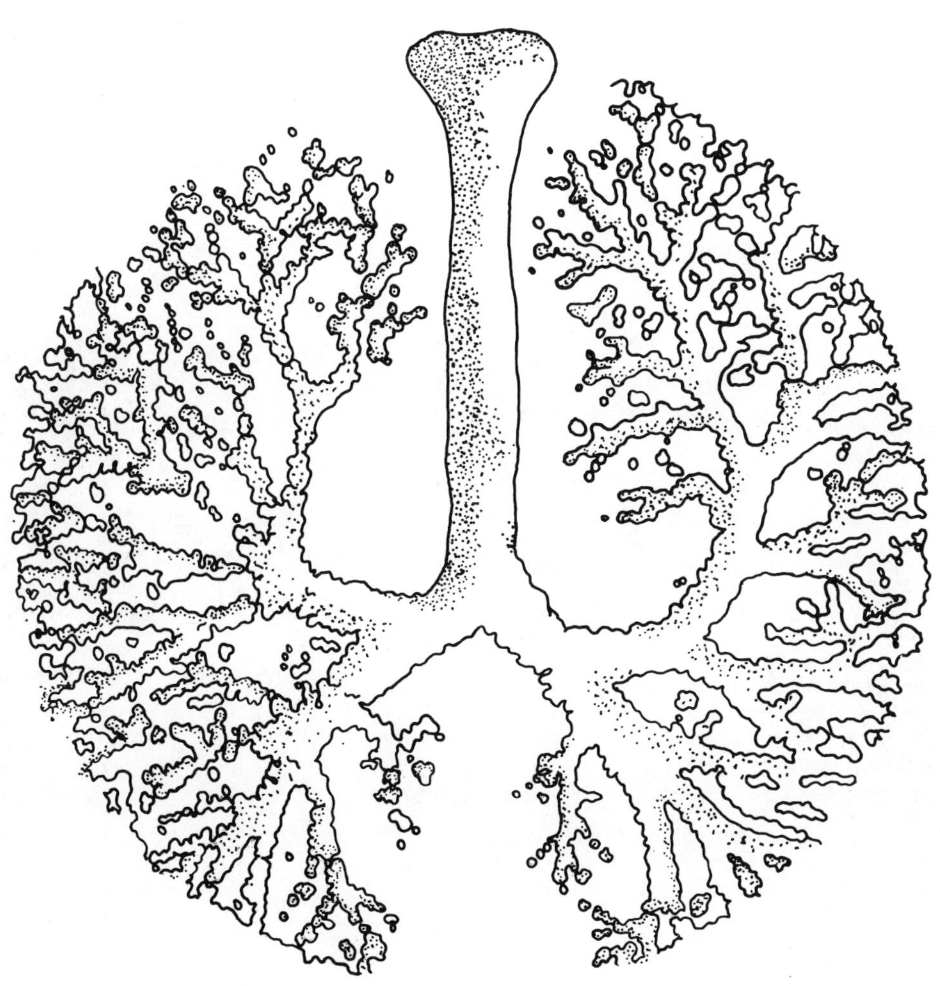

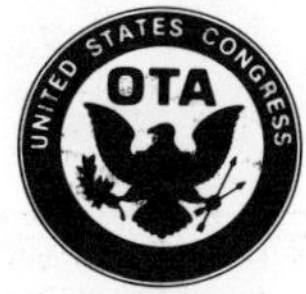

CONGRESS OF THE UNITED STATES
OFFICE OF TECHNOLOGY ASSESSMENT

For sale by the U.S. Government Printing Office
Superintendent of Documents, Mail Stop: SSOP, Washington, DC 20402-9328
ISBN 0-16-037923-7

Foreword

History reveals an enduring respect for lung function. In the biblical account of creation, man becomes a living soul when he receives the breath of life. Edward I of England banned the use of coal in 1273 because he found inhaling its smoke detrimental to human health. When asked how to ensure a long life, Sophie Tucker replied, "Keep breathing."

This Background Paper examines whether the agencies responsible for administering Federal environmental and health and safety laws have taken this concern for respiratory health to heart. Prepared at the request of the Senate Committee on Environment and Public Works and its Subcommittee on Toxic Substances, Environmental Oversight, Research and Development, the study describes technologies available to identify substances toxic to the lung and Federal efforts to control human exposure to such substances through regulatory and research programs. The analysis shows that new technologies hold great promise for revealing the potential adverse effects on the lung of new and existing substances, but that much remains to be learned. This Background Paper provides a partial response to the committees' request for an assessment of noncancer health risks in the environment and follows OTA's previous work on carcinogenic, neurotoxic, and immunotoxic substances.

OTA acknowledges the generous help of the workshop participants, reviewers, and contributors who gave their time to ensure the accuracy and completeness of this study. OTA, however, remains solely responsible for the contents of this Background Paper.

John H. Gibbons
Director

Workshop on Identifying and Controlling Pulmonary Toxicants, September 1991

Dr. Robert M. Friedman, *Workshop Chair*
Senior Associate
Oceans and Environment Program
Office of Technology Assessment

Dr. Margaret Becklake
Director, Respiratory Epidemiology Unit
McGill University

Dr. Arnold Brody
Head, Pulmonary Pathology
National Institute of Environmental
  Health Sciences

Dr. Daniel L. Costa
Chief, Pulmonary Toxicology Branch
Inhalation Toxicology Division
Health Effects Research Laboratory
U.S. Environmental Protection Agency

Dr. Joe L. Mauderly
Director
Inhalation Toxicology Research Institute
Lovelace Biomedical and Environmental
  Research Institute, Inc.

Dr. Roger O. McClellan
President
Chemical Industry Institute of Toxicology

Dr. Robert R. Mercer
Assistant Medical Research Professor
Department of Medicine
Duke University

Dr. Richard B. Schlesinger
Professor, Department of
  Environmental Medicine
New York University School of Medicine

Dr. Mark J. Utell
Director, Pulmonary and Critical
  Care Unit
University of Rochester Medical Center

Dr. Gregory Wagner
Director, Division of Respiratory
  Disease Studies
National Institute for Occupational
  Safety and Health

Dr. Ronald K. Wolff
Research Scientist
Lilly Research Laboratories

Note: OTA appreciates the valuable assistance and thoughtful critiques provided by the workshop participants. The participants do not, however, necessarily approve, disapprove, or endorse this background paper. OTA assumes full responsibility for the background paper and the accuracy of its contents.

Reviewers and Contributors

In addition to the workshop participants, OTA acknowledges the following individuals who reviewed drafts or otherwise contributed to this study.

Lois Adams
Office of Technology Assessment Liaison
Office of Legislative Affairs
U.S. Food and Drug Administration

Heinz W. Ahlers, J.D.
Division of Standards Development
  and Technology Transfer
National Institute for Occupational Safety
  and Health

John R. Balmes, M.D.
Assistant Professor of Medicine
Center for Occupational and Environmental Health
University of California, San Francisco

Rebecca Bascom, M.D.
Director, Environmental Research Facility
School of Medicine
University of Maryland

Robert P. Baughman, M.D.
Associate Professor of Medicine
Pulmonary/Critical Care Division
University of Cincinnati

Paul D. Blanc, M.D., M.S.P.H.
Assistant Professor of Medicine
Division of Occupational and
  Environmental Medicine
University of California-San Francisco

James C. Bonner, Ph.D.
Staff Fellow
Laboratory of Pulmonary Pathobiology
National Institute of Environmental Health Sciences

Carroll E. Cross, M.D.
Division of Pulmonary-Critical Care Medicine
Department of Internal Medicine
University of California-Davis Medical Center

Roger Detels, M.D., M.S.
Professor of Epidemiology
School of Public Health
University of California-Los Angeles

Fran Du Melle
Deputy Managing Director
American Lung Association

June Friedlander
Staff Specialist
National Institute for Occupational Safety
  and Health

Suzie Hazen
Director, 33/50 Program
Office of Air and Radiation
U.S. Environmental Protection Agency

Hillel S. Koren, Ph.D.
Acting Director
Human Studies Division
Health Effects Research Laboratory
U.S. Environmental Protection Agency

Martin Landry
Budget Analyst
Financial Management Office
National Institute for Occupational Safety
  and Health

John L. Mason, Ph.D.
Vice President
Engineering and Technology
Allied Signal Aerospace Co. (Ret.)

Barbara Packard, M.D., Ph.D.
Associate Director for Scientific
  Program Operations
National Heart, Lung, and Blood Institute

Jerry Phelps
Program Analyst
Office of Program Planning and Evaluation
Office of Director
National Institute of Environmental Health Sciences

William A. Pryor, Ph.D.
Director
Biodynamics Institute
Louisiana State University

Victor L. Roggli, M.D.
Associate Professor of Pathology
Department of Pathology
Duke University Medical Center

Robert Roth, Ph.D.
Professor
Department of Pharmacology and Toxicology
Michigan State University

Jonathan M. Samet, M.D.
Professor of Medicine
Medical Center
University of New Mexico

Anne P. Sassaman, Ph.D.
Director
Division of Extramural Research and Training
National Institute of Environmental Health Sciences

David A. Schwartz, M.D., M.P.H.
Director, Occupational Medicine
Pulmonary Disease Division
Department of Internal Medicine
University of Iowa

Joel Schwartz, Ph.D.
U.S. Environmental Protection Agency

Andrew Sivak, Ph.D.
President
Health Effects Institute

Frank E. Speizer, M.D.
Professor of Medicine and Environmental Science
School of Public Health
Harvard University

Jaro J. Vostal, M.D., Ph.D.
Environmental Activities Staff
General Motors Corp.

David B. Warheit, Ph.D.
Haskell Laboratory for Toxicology
  and Industrial Medicine
I.E. Du Pont De Nemours and Co.

Jane Warren, Ph.D.
Research Committee Director
Health Effects Institute

OTA Project Staff—Identifying and Controlling Pulmonary Toxicants

Roger C. Herdman, *Assistant Director, OTA*
Health and Life Sciences Division

Michael Gough, *Biological Applications Program Manager*

Holly L. Gwin, *Project Director*

Margaret McLaughlin, *Analyst*

Ellen Goode, *Research Assistant*

Katherine Kelly, *Contractor*

Desktop Publishing Specialists

Jene Lewis

Linda Rayford-Journiette

Carolyn Swann

Support Staff

Cecile Parker, *Office Administrator*

Contents

Boxes

Figures

Tables

Chapter 1

Introduction and Summary

Introduction and Summary

INTRODUCTION

Breathing sustains life. Each day an individual inhales between 10,000 and 20,000 liters of air. In the lungs, air releases oxygen to the bloodstream and picks up carbon dioxide and other waste products, which are then exhaled. Inhaled air contains many substances— naturally occurring and anthropogenic—other than oxygen. Some of these substances can injure the lungs and impede their function.

The potential for chemicals and materials used in industry, transportation, and households to be simultaneously beneficial and toxic to human life creates a legislative and regulatory dilemma. The challenge of balancing a strong economy, one that delivers products people need and desire, with the health and safety of the populace sometimes seems to be a tremendous burden.

Technological advances add to the weight of that burden. Thousands of new, potentially toxic substances enter the market annually. Advanced instruments help scientists measure the presence of new and existing substances in minute quantities. Substances formerly unknown or undetected suddenly become worrisome as technology provides the means to predict human risks from these substances.

Governmental concern that a substance might create an adverse health effect historically focused on carcinogenicity. Most Federal legislative and regulatory efforts to prevent or minimize human exposure to toxic substances have focused on identifying and controlling carcinogens. Physicians and researchers now recognize the noncancer, toxic effects of many substances. Some of these effects, for instance teratogenicity, have become the subject of specific legislative concern. Federal regulatory attention to other types of toxic injury (e.g., to the respiratory system, the immune system, the nervous system) depends on the more general mandate to protect human health. Some observers fear that historical emphasis on carcinogenicity, combined with limited agency resources, has led to neglect of noncancer health risks—risks that may be as widespread and severe as carcinogenicity.

The Senate Committee on Environment and Public Works, and its Subcommittee on Toxic Substances, Environmental Oversight, Research and Development, asked for assistance from the Office of Technology Assessment (OTA) in evaluating technologies to identify and control noncancer health risks in the environment. The committee's interests include advances in toxicology, research and testing programs in Federal agencies, and the consequences of exposure to toxic substances. OTA has published studies on neurotoxicity and immunotoxicity (18,19).

In further response to the committee's request, this background paper describes the state-of-the-art of identifying substances that can harm human lungs when inhaled. Chapter 2 provides a primer on human lung structure and function and describes lung diseases that have been associated with inhalation of toxic substances. Chapter 3 examines the technologies and methodologies used in laboratory, clinical, and epidemiologic studies to identify substances as toxic to the lung. Chapter 4 summarizes Federal research efforts and regulations designed to reduce human exposures to these substances.

SCOPE

This study assesses whether regulators using available toxicologic and epidemiologic investigative methods can obtain health effects data sufficient to identify airborne substances as pulmonary toxicants—substances toxic to the lung—when encountered at environmentally relevant exposure levels. Several terms within this description of the scope of work require definition to delineate the boundaries of OTA's inquiry.

Regulators—Regulators are the agencies, and their employees, with responsibility, under various environmental statutes, for setting standards to control human exposure to toxic substances. This study examines only Federal regulatory programs, but many States have environmental legislation and regulatory agendas that require the types of technologies and data discussed in this background paper.

Available toxicologic and epidemiologic investigative methods—This background paper reports on the technologies and methodologies applied in laboratory studies, human clinical studies, and field studies of human exposure (epidemiology) to determine whether substances exert toxic effects. As used in this study, the term laboratory studies comprises *in vitro* tests on cells, tissues, and fluids removed from animals and humans and *in vivo* tests on whole animals. The term human clinical studies refers to studies of the effects on humans of carefully controlled but purposeful exposures to potentially toxic substances; exposure to the suspected toxicant occurs in a clinical setting, hence the term. Epidemiologic studies are those in which investigators examine the effects on humans of exposures to suspected toxicants that occur without the intervention of the investigator and in a nonclinical setting, e.g., at home, in the workplace, at school, in the outdoors.

Airborne substances—Combustion, industrial processes, and other human activities can create inhalable gases and particles that may be toxic to the lungs. Technologies that enable assessment of the health effects of *inhaled* substances are the focus of this background paper. Substances taken orally (e.g., certain drugs) or absorbed through the skin (e.g., the pesticide paraquat) can be toxic to the human lung; some of the technologies discussed in this background paper could be used to identify their effects. However, this study limits itself to an examination of the technologies specifically applicable to investigation of the effects of airborne substances on the lung and the regulatory programs designed to control human exposure to such substances. The background paper discusses some biologic substances, e.g., organic dusts, but excludes consideration of infectious agents.

Environmentally relevant exposure levels—OTA defines "environmentally relevant exposure levels" as those that can reasonably be anticipated (under non-catastrophic circumstances) to occur in outdoor, residential, educational, commercial, and occupational environments in various regions of the United States.

This background paper describes a wide range of technologies that measure the biological effects of exposure to toxic substances—from technologies that identify minute changes in the cellular structure of the lung to technologies useful in the diagnosis of disease. Regulators use these technologies, singly or in combination, to determine not only whether a given dose of a suspected toxicant creates a measurable, biological effect but whether the measurable effect is itself adverse to respiratory health or correlates with development of an adverse condition. A definition for *adverse* remains a topic of considerable debate.

For example, scientists have developed several tests to detect decreases in lung function that result from exposure to toxic substances. While they agree on the technical capabilities of the tests, they disagree on the level of decreased function that should be deemed adverse for regulatory purposes. Using other tests, scientists are able to detect changes in the number of certain types of cells found in the lung following relatively low-level exposures to toxic substances. Given enough time and resources, scientists will be able to determine whether such changes reverse themselves, stabilize, or grow harmful under various types of exposure conditions. They will also learn whether those cellular changes actually impair lung function. Until those data are collected, however, regulators have insufficient evidence to deem the measurable effect adverse.

In this background paper, OTA describes the current technologies that measure the biological effects in the lung of toxic substances. The study also reports on Federal efforts to improve the technologies and regulate human exposures to substances deemed adverse. OTA makes no independent judgment concerning an appropriate definition of adverse effects or on the adequacy of current regulatory standards.

SUMMARY

This background paper distills some of the information available about the basic and applied sciences that enable the identification and control of pulmonary toxicants. More detailed reviews of lung structure and function, lung diseases, pulmonary toxicology, and epidemiology can be found in numerous sources (1,2,5,10,11,12). The following sections summarize much of the text that appears in subsequent chapters.

Lung Structure and Function

The lung comprises two of the three distinct regions of the human respiratory tract (figure 1-1). Air enters the body through the nose and mouth and passes through the *nasopharyngeal* region, where it is warmed and humidified. Air moves next through the *tracheobronchial* region (where the lung begins), which acts basically as a conducting passage. Finally air reaches the *pulmonary,* or *gas exchange,* region of the lung, where oxygen in the air is supplied to the blood, which delivers it to cells throughout the body. In turn, the blood releases a major waste product, carbon dioxide (CO_2), and other gaseous components and metabolites to air remaining in the lung, which is exhaled. The pulmonary region has a tremendous surface area—in adults about the size of a single's tennis court—which permits efficient gas exchange (oxygen for CO_2).

The respiratory system is equipped with defense mechanisms. The nasopharyngeal region can filter large particles and absorb gases with high water solubility before they reach the lung. Cells that line the tracheobronchial region secrete mucus that traps inhaled particles and reactive gases, and other cells sweep the mucus up and out of the respiratory system to the digestive system. Certain cells that reside in the pulmonary region can ingest and destroy particles that penetrate to that region. Some toxic substances can bypass or overwhelm these defense mechanisms, resulting in lung injury or disease.

Lung Injury and Disease

Lung function suffers when resistance to airflow in the conducting airways (tracheobronchial region) increases or when a loss of healthy surface area in the pulmonary region prevents transfer of sufficient amounts of oxygen to the blood. Many agents—manmade and natural, physical and biological—can cause these basic problems, which are characteristic of several forms of disabling lung diseases (e.g., asthma, fibrosis, emphysema). Because of the limited types of pulmonary responses and the large number of agents to which individuals are exposed, the association of individual agents with specific responses has been difficult. Careful observation and experimentation over the years, however, has led to conclusions about the potential of certain toxicants to cause or exacerbate lung diseases.

Several outdoor air pollutants, e.g., sulfur dioxide, increase the breathing difficulties of high-risk groups (e.g., asthmatics). Tobacco smoke causes cancer (beyond the scope of this report), chronic bronchitis, and emphysema, and contributes to an increased incidence of respiratory disease in children of smoking parents, which may lead to chronic lung problems as they age. Occupational exposure to inhaled chemicals and fibers has yielded some of the strongest evidence linking toxic substances to lung disease.

Many tools for studying the toxicity of airborne substances have been developed in recent years, but the number of toxicants to be assessed and the amount of data required to substantiate their toxicity present a challenging task to toxicologists, epidemiologists, and regulators. Studies are under way to determine whether persistent human lung problems are correlated with exposures to many of the gases and particles encountered in everyday life.

Pulmonary Toxicology and Epidemiology

Investigators use three, complementary lines of research to assess the effects on the lung of inhaled pollutants: laboratory studies, including in vitro tests and tests in whole animals, human clinical studies, and epidemiology. Each type of study has strengths and weaknesses. In in vitro tests, scientists examine the

Figure 1-1—The Human Respiratory Tract

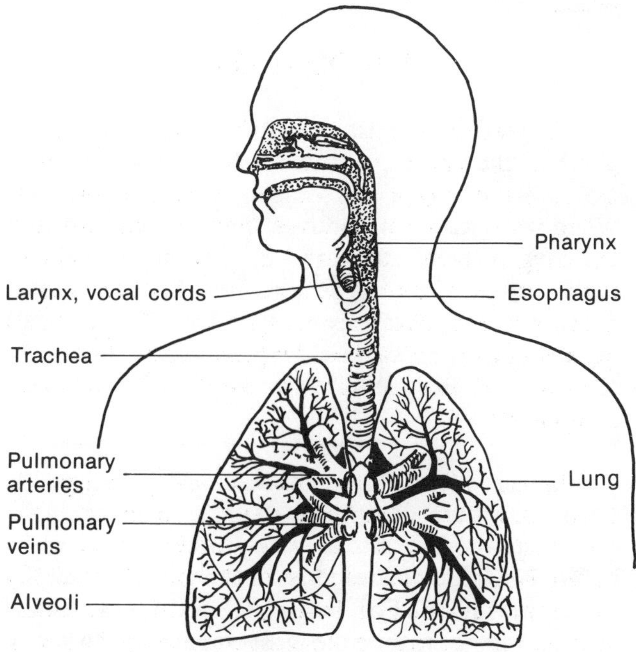

SOURCE: Office of Technology Assessment, 1992.

structure or functional capability of tissues and cells to determine the effects of toxic exposures. These studies are informative but may not give a complete picture of a toxicant's effects. In in vivo studies, scientists use animals whose respiratory systems resemble the human system and attempt to mimic expected human exposure conditions as closely as possible. Such studies are useful but are limited by the difficulty in extrapolating results from animals to humans. Clinical studies allow careful control of exposure conditions and provide human data. However, they are restricted to relatively brief exposures that will create no lasting injury and, like most animal studies, are limited to exposures to one or two substances at a time rather than the complex mixtures actually encountered in the environment. Epidemiologic studies analyze the effects created by toxicants under actual exposure conditions but are limited by imprecise measurements of exposure to the toxicant under study and by confounding factors such as smoking, preexisting disease, and unknown effects of other exposures.

Whether involving animals or humans, studies employ functional, structural, or biochemical methods of investigation. Functional assays measure the mechanics of breathing, decreases or increases in gas-exchange capacity, and the ability of the lungs to rid themselves of foreign particles, among other things. Structural studies employ the traditional techniques of pathology to gather substantial information about pulmonary toxicity. Prepared slices of excised lungs can be examined with microscopes for evidence of alterations in structure. Various regions of the excised lung can be examined for the presence of particles. Cells can be examined for injury. Advances in cellular biology in recent years contributed to some of the most important new methods of pulmonary toxicology. Toxicologists using biochemical methods can now study the cellular interactions and biochemical mechanisms of the lung using fluids recovered from lungs. In addition to biological tests on an exposed population, epidemiologists can use various databases, including mortality and morbidity statistics, hospital admissions records, and diaries of respiratory symptoms, to correlate exposure to toxicants with lung injury and disease.

In the laboratory and clinic, investigators can control the amount of the substance under study delivered to the test subject and can exclude all other exposures. The technologies used produce precise measurements of exposure but cannot reproduce the actual exposure conditions people encounter in their daily lives. Epidemiologists cannot control the dose of a toxicant received by their study subjects, but advances in stationary and personal exposure monitoring technologies have improved the accuracy of exposure measurements in epidemiologic studies. All scientists studying the effects of pulmonary toxicants must consider the fact that *exposure*—the amount of a toxicant found in the inhalable air—frequently differs from *biologically effective dose*—the amount of toxicant actually retained in the lung for sufficient time to cause problems. Differences in human and animal lungs have a major impact on biologically effective dose and create many of the difficulties in extrapolating test results from animals to humans.

Integrated use of laboratory, clinical, and epidemiologic techniques often produces the best results. For instance, increased respiratory symptoms in a working population exposed to chemical fumes might suggest the need for laboratory studies of the chemical's health effects. Following the laboratory experiments, clinical studies might be performed to obtain more accurate data about harmful and harmless levels of short-term exposure in humans. Once a permissible exposure level is established for the workplace, workers could be monitored, in an epidemiologic study, to determine whether long-term exposures created effects that did not show up in the short-term studies. Pulmonary toxicologists, clinicians, and epidemiologists share the objective of identifying the health effects of airborne substances to which humans are or will likely be exposed.

AIR QUALITY

Air comprises those gases that form the atmosphere of the earth. At altitudes below 80 kilometers molecular nitrogen and oxygen dominate the mix. When water vapor is removed from the air, nitrogen and oxygen constitute 78 and 21 percent (by volume) of the air, respectively. The remaining 1 percent of this dry air consists principally of argon, but CO_2 and small quantities of neon, helium, krypton, xenon, hydrogen, methane and nitrous oxide are also found as constant components of air.

Human activities (agriculture, industry, transportation) contribute additional, variable components—pollutants—to the mix of gases called air. Level of industrialization creates most of the global variability in air pollution. For instance, wood (and other biomass) smoke may be the most common pollutant in nonindustrialized countries, while fossil fuel combustion byproducts (e.g., sulfur oxides, nitrogen oxides, particulate matter) constitute the major air pollutants in heavily industrialized countries. Regional differences in pollutants depend on population, activity mix, geography, and climatic conditions. Within a community, air quality may differ significantly upwind and downwind of, for instance, a power plant. Family members may experience quite different pollutant exposure conditions depending on how much time they spend at work, school, or home.

In the United States, fossil fuel combustion contributes to both major types of outdoor air pollution—chemically reducing pollution and chemically oxidizing, or photochemical, pollution. Reducing type pollution is characterized by sulfur dioxide and fossil fuel smoke and by conditions of fog and cool temperatures. This type of pollution occurs mainly in the eastern part of the country, primarily in the Mid-Atlantic and Northeastern States. Oxidizing type pollution is characterized by hydrocarbons, oxides of nitrogen, and photochemical oxidants and results from the action of sunlight on polluted air masses. This pollution problem, infamous in several western U.S. cities (e.g., Los Angeles), now strikes the northeast and southeast in the summer months as well. Other types of pollutants pose seasonal problems, for instance woodsmoke in certain cities during the winter months. Toxic pollutants emitted from industrial sites or from hazardous waste sites can present highly localized air quality problems (see table 1-1). Outdoor air pollution is regulated under the Clean Air Act and other environmental statutes.

Some occupations involve significant potential for exposure to airborne toxicants. These types of exposures generally are regulated under the Occupational Safety and Health Act and the Federal Mine Safety and Health Act. Health and safety regulations have reduced many of the acute exposure problems experienced by workers; experts are uncertain whether

Table 1-1—The Seventeen Chemicals of the 33/50 Program, 1989

Chemicals	Total releases and transfers (pounds)	Total air releases and transfers (pounds)	Industry
Cadmium and compounds*	1,147,783	119,841	Primary metals
Chromium and compounds*	64,284,382	2,238,473	Chemicals
Lead and compounds	54,371,117	2,449,799	Primary metals
Mercury and compounds*	216,433	29,239	Chemicals
Nickel and compounds*	22,342,311	1,128,788	Primary metals
Benzene*	28,591,407	24,683,026	Primary metals
Methyl ethyl ketone*	156,992,642	127,631,835	Plastics
Methyl isobutyl ketone	38,849,703	30,682,832	Chemicals
Toluene	322,521,176	255,437,878	Chemicals
Xylenes (mixed isomers)*	185,442,035	147,486,804	Transport
Carbon tetrachloride	4,607,809	3,367,248	Chemicals
Chloroform (Trichloromethane)	27,325,508	24,268,093	Paper
Methylchloride (Dichloromethane)*	130,355,581	109,272,003	Chemicals
Tetrachloroethylene (Perchloroethylene)*	30,058,581	25,504,477	Transport
1, 1, 1-Trichloroethane (Methyl chloroform)*	185,026,191	168,617,910	Transport
Trichloroethylene*	48,976,806	44,325,687	Fabricated metals
Cyanides	11,976,370	[a]	Chemicals

*EPA notes a respiratory effect.

[a]Cyanide emissions to the air have been estimated to be in excess of 44 million pounds per year. The largest single source of air emissions is vehicle exhaust, which accounts for over 90 percent of this total. This type of emission is not reported under the EPA's Toxic Release Inventory National Report.

SOURCE: U.S. Environmental Protection Agency, Office of Toxic Substances, Economics and Technology Division, *Toxics in the Community: National and Local Perspectives - The 1989 Toxics Release Inventory National Report,* EPA-560/4-91-014 (Washington, DC: September 1991).

current exposure limits prevent the types of persistent problems that might be associated with long-term, low-level exposures.

Most people spend most of their time indoors—at home, at school, or in the office. The primary indoor air pollutants are tobacco smoke, nitrogen dioxide, carbon monoxide, woodsmoke, biological agents (e.g., molds, animal dander), formaldehyde, various volatile organic compounds, and radon. Indoor pollutants may be generated by personal activities, such as cigarette smoking, or by things outside an individual's control, such as the geological formation on which a house sits, the source of radon. Indoor, airborne toxicants are important sources of individual exposure to toxicants that may appear in the outdoor air as well (e.g., nitrogen dioxide) and should be considered in health effects assessments. Outside of certain occupational settings, exposures to indoor, airborne toxicants remain largely unregulated.

Airborne gases and particles emanate from multiple indoor and outdoor sources, and individuals experience multiple exposures to airborne toxicants as they go about their lives. The mix of substances individuals inhale and the variety of circumstances under which they do it makes it very hard for scientists and policymakers to sort out the effects of specific substances. Some individuals are more susceptible than others to the effects of airborne toxicants, which makes it difficult for regulators to determine acceptable levels of exposure once the effects of specific substances have been determined. The technologies of air quality measurement, exposure assessment, and toxicological testing contribute to better risk assessment and better policymaking, but currently leave many uncertainties in their wake.

CONCLUSIONS

Scientists and regulators have a high degree of confidence in existing laboratory, clinical, and epidemiologic methods for studying the adverse effects of acute (short-term, high-level) exposures to existing chemicals and particles. When analyzing acute responses, scientists isolate the effects of a specific substance in

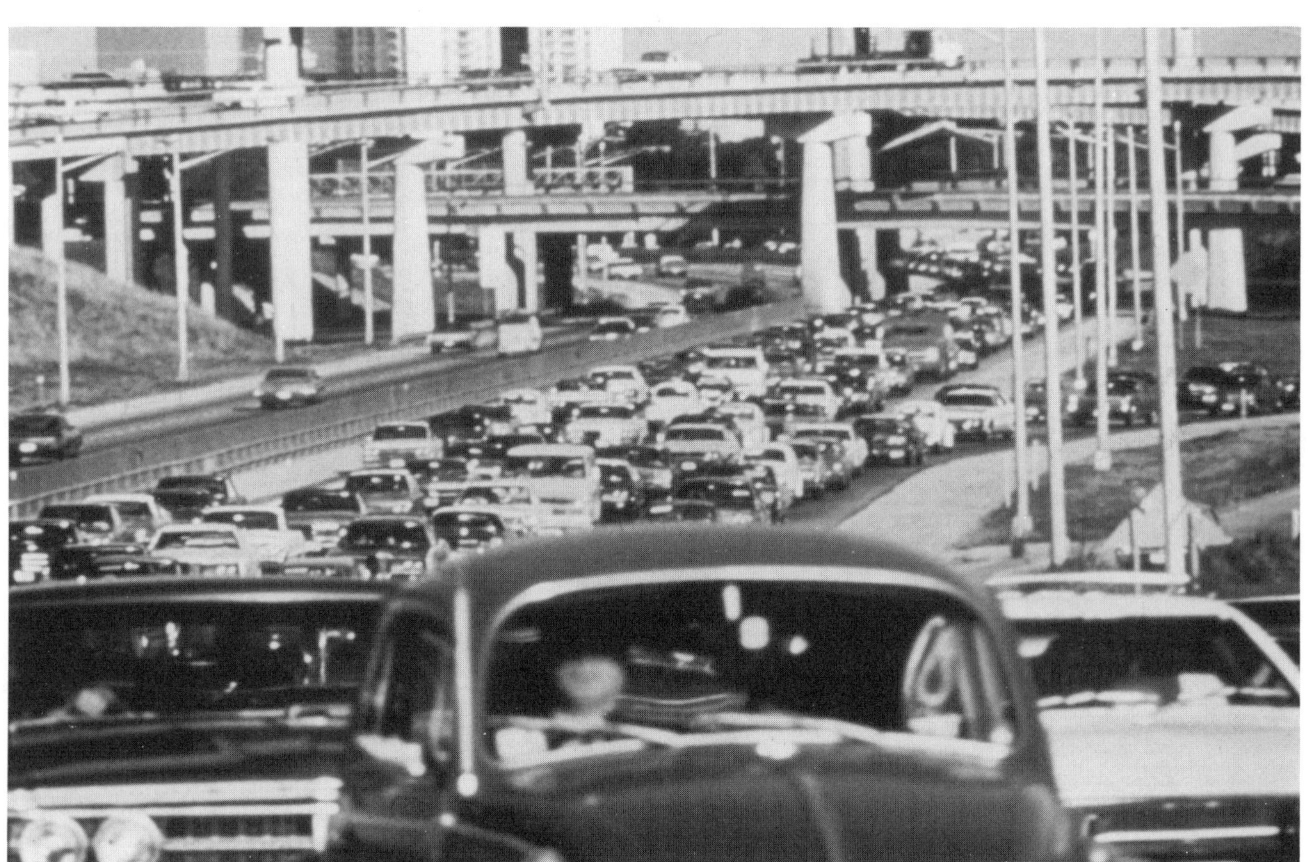

Photo credit: South Coast Air Quality Management District, El Monte, CA.

animal studies using controlled exposure conditions and then couple those test results with information (when available) about the real-life experience of exposed humans. This method enables relatively clear association between exposure to a specific substance and specific health effects, though evidence can still be equivocal. Analysis of the effects of chronic exposure is under way for many substances and data can readily be acquired from animal studies (given time and resources). However, credible human data on the effects of chronic exposure are more difficult to obtain because of extraneous factors that can affect study results (e.g., difficulties in determining the effects of previous exposures; opportunities for exposure to multiple substances). Where substances are regulated because of their pulmonary toxicity, the regulations are primarily based on health effects observed following acute exposures.

A synopsis of the attempt to set a standard for ozone that prevents adverse health effects illuminates the power and limitations of current technologies within the current regulatory framework for protection of public health. Ozone is produced when its precursors, volatile organic compounds (VOC's) and nitrogen oxides (NO_x), combine in the presence of sunlight. Current EPA regulations require States to maintain ozone concentrations in the air below 0.12 ppm. Areas where ozone in the ambient air exceeds a peak 1-hour average concentration of 0.12 ppm more than 1 day per year (averaged over 3 years) are labeled nonattainment areas and are subject to legal sanctions (17).

EPA adopted the current standard for ozone exposure on the basis of evidence of the health effects of short-term exposures slightly above that level. At the time the standard was set, scientists agreed that short-term exposures to ozone caused reductions in lung function and increases in respiratory symptoms, airway reactivity, permeability, and inflammation in the general population. Asthmatics were known to suffer additional effects, including increased rates of medication usage and restricted activities (9).

The database on ozone's health effects has continued to grow since EPA set the standard for exposure in 1979. Data from human clinical studies now show that lung function decreases during exposure to 0.12 ppm (the current regulatory standard) and continues to decrease during constant exposures of 6 hours or more (4,6). Biochemical studies on lung fluids removed from individuals who were exercising during exposure to

ozone above, at, and below the current regulatory standard showed lung inflammation (8,9).

The acute effects of exposure to ozone have also been the subject of epidemiologic studies. Lung function in children engaged in outdoor recreation activities decreased during exposure to ozone, and outdoor exposure caused a greater decrease than clinical exposure at the same concentration of ozone, indicating that other substances in the outdoor air potentiated the response to ozone (15,16). School children showed similar responses in another study (7).

Researchers have begun to study the effects of chronic exposure to ozone in various populations. A study of residents in the Los Angeles area showed that chronic exposure to oxidant pollution affects baseline lung function (3). Another study from the Los Angeles area, this time on the autopsied lungs of young accident victims, showed structural abnormalities in the lungs that were not expected in individuals of that age range (13). An analysis of pulmonary function data collected in a national survey showed a clear association between reduced lung function and annual average ozone concentrations in excess of 0.04 ppm (14). Based on epidemiologic research findings, a growing number of scientists believes that chronic exposure to ozone may cause premature aging of the lung, and they find support for this opinion in recent studies on rats and monkeys (9).

Scientists disagree on the health significance of the decreased lung function measured in the human clinical studies (9). EPA's Clean Air Science Advisory Committee (CASAC) split when asked to reach closure concerning a scientifically supportable upper bound for a 1-hour ozone standard, with half the members accepting the current standard and half recommending a reduction in permissible exposure levels (20). CASAC noted that "resolution of the adverse health effect issue represents a blending of scientific and policy judgments." Little information on the human health effects of chronic ozone exposures has been available to regulators or their advisors, and scientists continue to urge that results from such studies be assessed cautiously. Despite strong evidence that ozone is harmful to human health at currently allowable exposure concentrations (9,21), EPA has not proposed a revision of the ozone standard.

Regulators face greater difficulties when developing supportable exposure standards for substances with smaller health effects databases or with databases limited to results of laboratory studies (as with new substances). The difficulties lie in the technologies themselves (e.g., remaining uncertainties regarding extrapolating results from animals to humans) and in balancing competing interests (e.g., dependence on automobiles versus air pollutants' harmful effects).

None of the technologies currently in use or under development for assessing pulmonary toxicity promises to be a near term alternative to extensive (costly) studies involving animals and humans. Scientists studying the behavior of gases and particles in the lungs of various animal species and humans hold out hope for continued improvements in techniques for extrapolation from animal studies to humans. Researchers investigating the mechanisms of disease believe what they discover may enable extrapolation from study results on existing chemicals to the likely effects of new substances with similar physical properties. At present, however, there is no scientific agreement that the effects measured by new toxicologic methods are adverse—distinctly and permanently harmful—instead of changes that may evince the recuperative properties of the lung. Therefore regulators can only continue to balance the costs and benefits of different regulatory levels rather than choose a regulatory level for pulmonary toxicants that will clearly avoid adverse human health effects.

CHAPTER 1 REFERENCES

1. Amdur, M.O., Doull, J., and Klaassen, C.D. (eds.), *Casarett and Doull's Toxicology: The Basic Science of Poisons, 4th ed.* (Elmsford, NY: Pergamon Press, 1991).
2. Crystal, R.G., and West, J.B. (eds.), *The Lung: Scientific Foundations* (New York, NY: Raven Press, 1991).
3. Detels, R., Tashkin, D.P., Sayre, J.W., et al., "The UCLA Population Studies of Chronic Obstructive Respiratory Disease. 9. Lung Function Changes Associated With Chronic Exposure to Photochemical Oxidants: A Cohort Study Among Never-Smokers," *Chest* 92(4):594-603, October 1987.
4. Folinsbee, L.J., McDonnell, W.F., and Horstman, D.H., "Pulmonary Function and Symptom Responses After 6.6 Hour Exposure to 0.12 ppm Ozone With Moderate Exercise," *Journal of the Air Pollution Control Association* 38:28-35, January 1988.
5. Gardner, D.E., Crapo, J.D., and Massaro, E.J. (eds.), *Toxicology of the Lung* (New York, NY: Raven Press, 1988).
6. Horstman, D.H., Folinsbee, L.J., Ives, P.J., et al., "Ozone Concentration and Pulmonary Response Relationships for 6.6-Hour Exposures With Five Hours of Moderate Exercise to 0.08, 0.10, and 0.12 ppm," *American Review of Respiratory Disease* 142(5):1158-1163, November 1990.
7. Kinney, P.L., Ware, J.H., and Spengler, J.D., "A Critical Evaluation of Acute Ozone Epidemiology Results," *Archives of Environmental Health* 43(2):168-73, March/April 1988.
8. Koren, H.S., Devlin, R.B., Graham, D.E., et al., "Ozone-Induced Inflammation in the Lower Airways of Human Subjects," *American Review of Respiratory Disease* 139:407-415, 1989.
9. Lippmann, M., "Health Effects of Tropospheric Ozone," *Environmental Science and Technology* 25(12):1954-1962, December 1991.
10. McClellan, R.O., and Henderson, R.F. (eds.), *Concepts in Inhalation Toxicology* (New York, NY: Hemisphere Publishing Corp., 1989).
11. National Research Council, Committee on the Epidemiology of Air Pollutants, *Epidemiology and Air Pollution* (Washington, DC: National Academy Press, 1985).
12. National Research Council, Subcommittee on Pulmonary Toxicology, *Biologic Markers in Pulmonary Toxicology* (Washington, DC: National Academy Press, 1989).
13. Sherwin, R.P., and Richters, V., "Centriacinar Region (CAR) Disease in the Lungs of Young Adults: A Preliminary Report," in *Tropospheric Ozone and the Environment* (Pittsburgh, PA: Air and Waste Management Association, 1991.)
14. Schwartz, J., "Lung Function and Chronic Exposure to Air Pollution: A Cross-Sectional Analysis of NHANES II," *Environmental Research* 50(2):309-321, December 1989.
15. Spektor, D.M., Lippmann, M., Lioy, P.J., et al., "Effects of Ambient Ozone on Respiratory Function in Active, Normal Children" *American Review of Respiratory Disease* 137:313-320, 1988.
16. Spektor, D.M., Thurston, G.D., Mao, J., et al., "Effects of Single- and Multiday Ozone Exposure on Respiratory Function in Active Normal Children," *Environmental Research* 55(2):107-122, August 1991.
17. U.S. Congress, Office of Technology Assessment, *Catching Our Breath: Next Steps for Reducing Urban Ozone,* OTA-O-412 (Washington, DC: U.S. Government Printing Office, July 1989).

18. U.S. Congress, Office of Technology Assessment, *Neurotoxicity: Identifying and Controlling Poisons of the Nervous System*, OTA-BA-436 (Washington, DC: U.S. Government Printing Office, April 1990).

19. U.S. Congress, Office of Technology Assessment, *Identifying and Controlling Immunotoxic Substances—Background Paper,* OTA-BP-BA-75 (Washington, DC: U.S. Government Printing Office, April 1991).

20. U.S. Environmental Protection Agency, Clean Air Scientific Advisory Committee, *Review of the NAAQS for Ozone,* EPA-SAB-CASAC-89-1092 (Washington, DC: U.S. Environmental Protection Agency, 1989).

21. Van Bree, L., Lioy, P.J., Rombout, P.J., et al., "A More Stringent and Longer-Term Standard for Tropospheric Ozone: Emerging New Data on Health Effects and Potential Exposure," *Toxicology and Applied Pharmacology* 103(3):377-382, May 1990.

The Respiratory System and Its Response to Harmful Substances

The Respiratory System and Its Response To Harmful Substances

INTRODUCTION

People can live for days without food or water, but if they stop breathing, they die within minutes. The apparatus of breathing—the respiratory system—supplies a critical component of life, oxygen, and disposes of a major waste product, carbon dioxide. To supply the amount of oxygen required for survival, the respiratory system must be capable of handling between 10,000 and 20,000 liters of air per day.

The air that enters the respiratory system contains many substances other than oxygen, including natural constituents (e.g., nitrogen) and human contributions (e.g., fossil fuel combustion byproducts). Various defense mechanisms of the respiratory system eliminate the unnatural components of air from the body and repair any damage they do. But exposure to large amounts of toxic substances or chronic exposure to lower levels can overwhelm the ability of the respiratory system to protect and repair itself, sometimes resulting in impaired lung function.

This chapter describes the structure and function of the respiratory system and some of the ways the respiratory system protects itself against harmful substances. It then briefly describes major diseases associated with exposure to toxic substances. This chapter does not cover the effects of exposure to radiation or infectious agents, nor does it describe lung cancer. More detailed descriptions of the respiratory system and respiratory diseases are presented elsewhere (7,13,26,28,29).

STRUCTURE AND FUNCTION OF THE RESPIRATORY SYSTEM

Air enters the body through the nose and mouth and moves through the major airways to deeper portions of the lungs (figure 2-1). There oxygen can pass across thin membranes to the bloodstream. Each region of the respiratory system is made of specialized cells that work together to transport air, keep the lung clean, defend it against harmful or infectious agents,

Figure 2-1—The Human Respiratory Tract

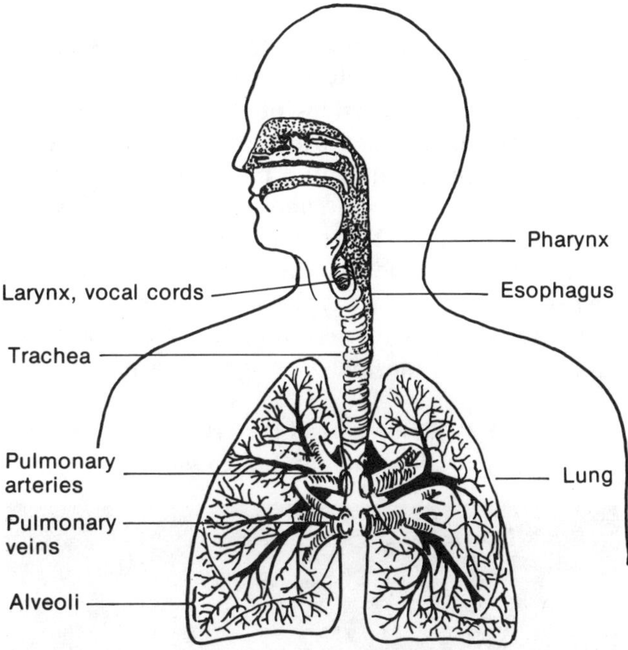

SOURCE: Office of Technology Assessment, 1992.

and provide a thin, large surface for the exchange of oxygen and carbon dioxide.

Upper Respiratory Tract

The upper airways begin at the nose and mouth and extend through the pharynx to the larynx. This nasophoryngeal region is lined with ciliated cells and mucous membranes that warm and humidify the air and remove some particles. Gases that are very water soluble are also absorbed readily by the mucus in this part of the respiratory tract, protecting the more delicate tissues deeper in the respiratory tract from the effects of exposure to such gases.

The Tracheobronchial Tree

After passing through the larynx, air flows through the trachea, or windpipe. The trachea divides into two bronchi which carry air into the two lungs. The bronchi subdivide repeatedly into smaller and smaller bronchi and then into bronchioles, which also successively divide and narrow (figure 2-2). The smallest bronchioles, found at the end of the tracheobronchial region, are less than a millimeter in diameter.

The Pulmonary Region

In the pulmonary region, the bronchioles divide into alveolar ducts and alveolar sacs. Budding from the walls of these last portions of the airways are tiny, cup-like chambers called alveoli (figure 2-3). The alveoli are only one-quarter of a millimeter in diameter (just barely visible to the unaided eye) and have extremely thin walls. Their outer surface is covered by a dense network of fine blood vessels, or capillaries. Gas exchange occurs when oxygen diffuses from the space inside an alveolus through its lining fluid, past the alveolar membrane and its supporting membrane,

Figure 2-2—Branching of the Tracheobronchial Region (Human Lung Cast)

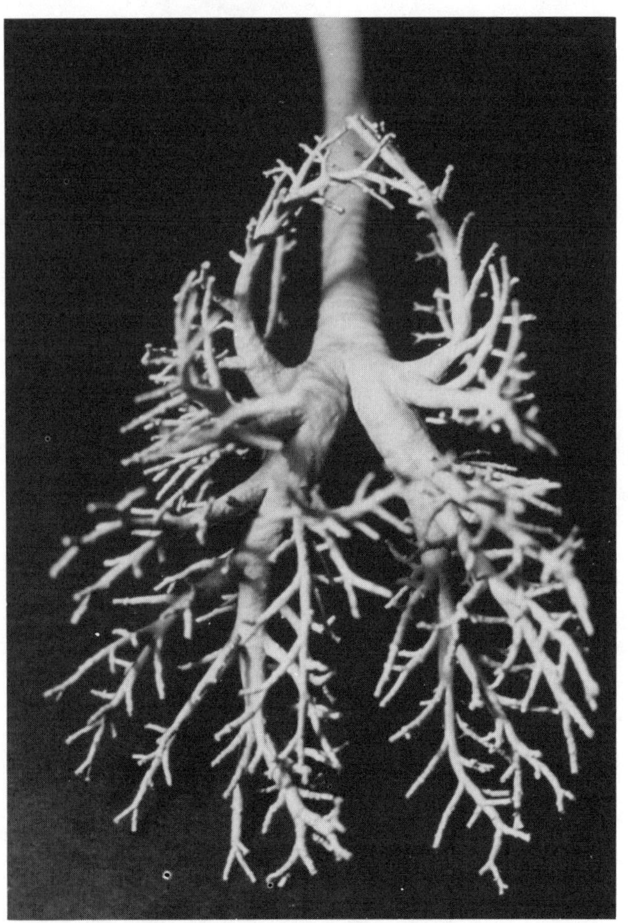

Photo credit: D. Costa, Environmental Protection Agency

Figure 2-3—Alveoli

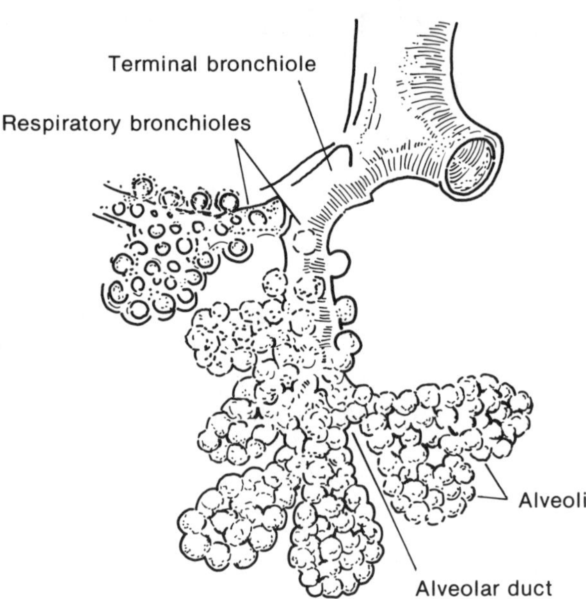

SOURCE: Office of Technology Assessment, 1992.

through the space between the alveolus and the capillary ("the interstitial space"), and finally across the membranes of the capillary. Carbon dioxide diffuses in the opposite direction, from the red blood cells in the capillaries to the space inside the alveolus (figure 2-4).

The adult human lung contains approximately 300 million alveoli. Taken together, the alveoli give the human lung a huge internal surface, about 70 square meters. This large area allows for enough oxygen to diffuse into the blood to supply the body's needs, but it also exposes a very large, thin-walled area, about the size of a single tennis court, to toxic substances inhaled in the air.

The Pulmonary Circulation

Oxygen diffuses from the alveoli into the blood in the capillaries. Red blood cells contain a specialized protein, hemoglobin, which can reversibly bind molecules of oxygen. The heart pumps the blood to the rest of the body. Deep within the tissues, the oxygen is released to be used by cells in generating energy. As the body's cells use oxygen, they produce carbon dioxide. Veins carry blood from body tissues back to the right side of the heart, which pumps blood to the pulmonary capillaries to be oxygenated again. Carbon dioxide diffuses from the capillaries into the alveoli and is exhaled.

Figure 2-4—Gas Exchange in the Pulmonary Region

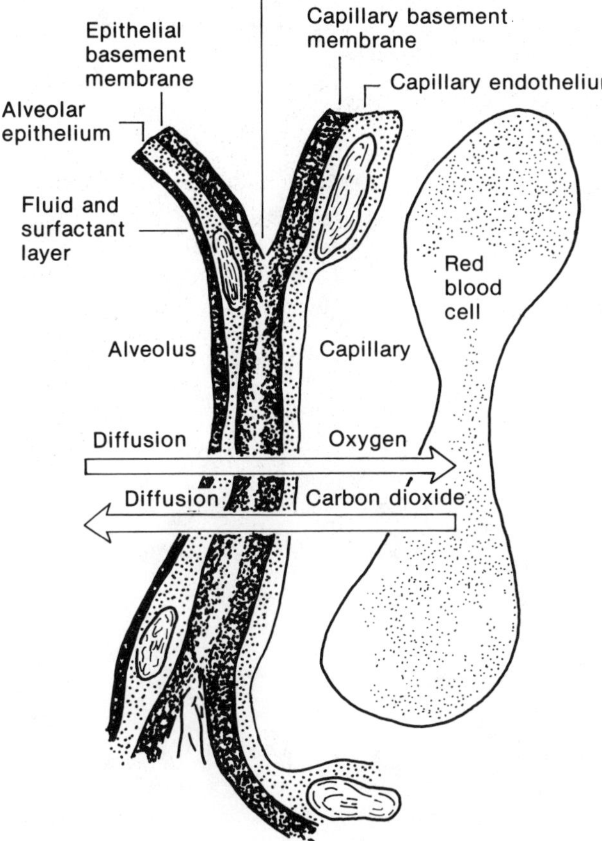

SOURCE: Office of Technology Assessment, 1992.

The Pleural Cavity

The lungs are contained within the chest cavity, but are not attached to the wall of the chest. The pleural space that separates the lungs from the chest wall contains a small amount of fluid and is bounded by membranes called the pleura. This arrangement allows the lungs to move freely in the chest, permitting full expansion.

During inhalation, the muscles in the rib cage and the diaphragm, a dome-shaped muscle beneath the lungs, contract. As the diaphragm contracts, it flattens, increasing the space in the chest. The ribs lift, further increasing the space for the lungs to expand. As the chest expands, the pressure within the lungs falls below atmospheric pressure, and air is drawn into the lungs, inflating them. As the muscles relax, air is exhaled, and the lungs deflate. The rate of respiration changes in response to physical and mental conditions, such as sleep, exercise, or changes in altitude.

Cells of the Respiratory System

The respiratory system contains over 40 different types of cells. Each cell type performs function important for efficient gas exchange.

A continuous sheet of cells forms a membrane, called the epithelium, lining the airways. Healthy epithelium contains few or no gaps, so water, ions, or other substances that cross the epithelium must pass through cells. The specific permeability properties of the cells control the rate at which substances, such as inhaled pollutants, cross the epithelium.

Interspersed among the cells that make up the surface of the lining of the airways are a variety of secretory cells. These secrete mucus which traps dust and other particles. Most of the cells of the epithelium have microscopic hair-like structures on their surface called cilia (figure 2-5). The cilia beat rhythmically, brushing the mucus and particles trapped in it up to the pharynx where they are usually swallowed unnoticed and pass out of the body through the digestive system.

Different types of cells make up the lining of the alveoli. The area of the lining consists primarily of Type I cells, which are very thin and spread over a relatively large area. The lining also includes the Type II cells. Type II cells are more numerous, but because of their more rounded shape, they make up only about 7 percent of the area of the lining of the aveoli. The Type II cells release proteins and lipids that provide a thin, fluid lining for the inside of the alveoli. The fluid protects the delicate Type I cells and reduces the surface tension in the alveoli, preventing collapse of the alveoli under pressure.

The alveoli also contain macrophages, specialized defense cells that move freely over the surface of an alveolus (figure 2-5). Macrophages ingest foreign particles by a process called phagocytosis. During phagocytosis, a macrophage extends flaps to form a membrane-bound pocket around a foreign body. The macrophage releases enzymes into the pocket that can break down many foreign particles, especially organic materials. The breakdown products may be released or absorbed by the cell. Foreign matter that is not organic often cannot be broken down and may remain stored

Figure 2-5—Ciliated Cells and Alveolar Macrophages

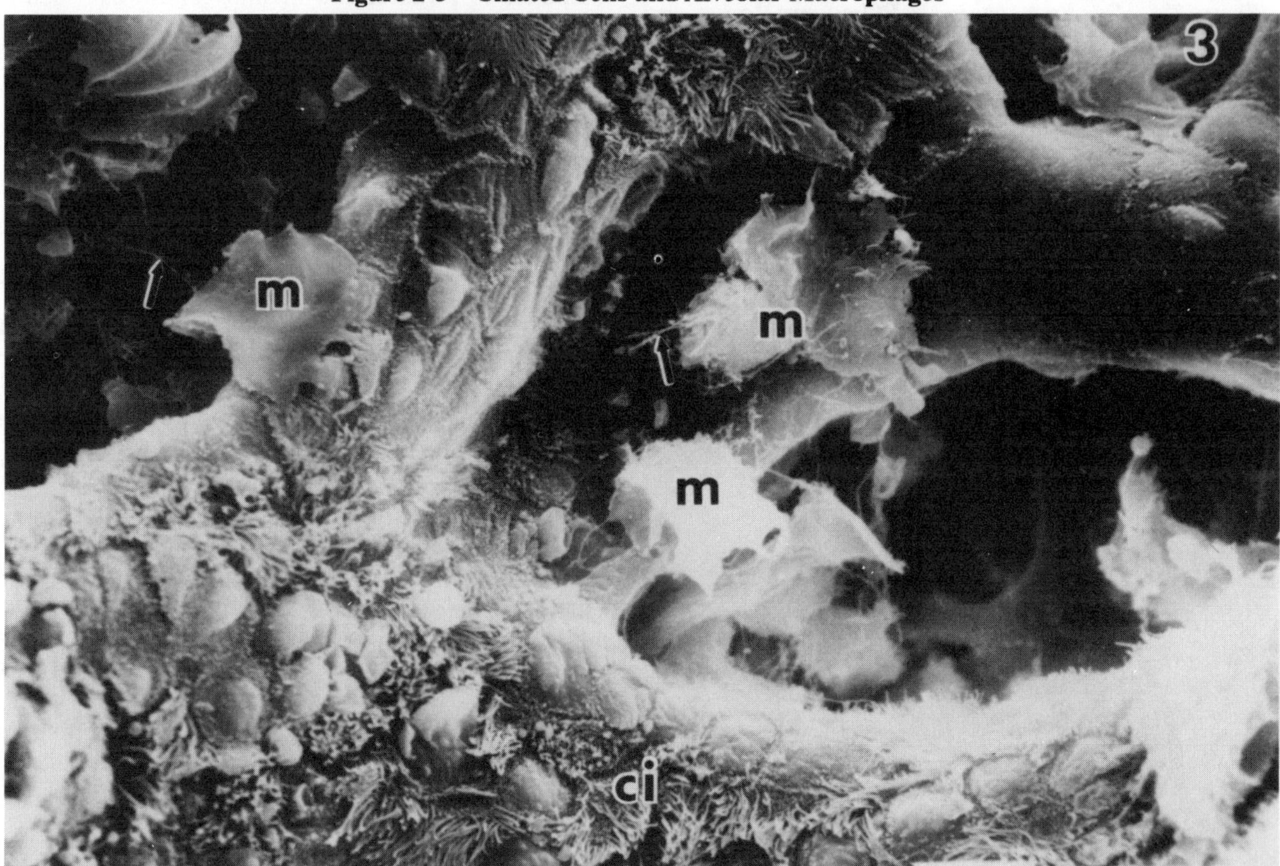

Photo credit: A. Brody, National Institute of Environmental Health Sciences

This photograph shows ciliated cells (ci) and alveolar macrophages (m) at the bronchiolar- alveolar duct junction. The arrows mark the presence of asbestos fibers.

in intracellular compartments. In addition to phagocytosis of foreign substances, macrophages also play important roles in immune responses in the lung.

The capillaries that surround the alveoli are also lined by a continuous sheet of cells, the endothelium. Unlike the lining of the airways, the endothelial lining of the capillaries is slightly leaky, allowing some exchange of water and solutes between the blood and the interstitial fluid.

The interstitial space, the small area separating alveoli from surrounding capillaries, contains cells of the immune system. It also contains fibroblasts, cells that produce fibers of collagen and elastin that form an elaborate network to provide a mechanical support system for the lung. Collagen fibers are very strong but cannot stretch much; elastin fibers are not as strong but can be stretched considerably before breaking. These collagen and elastin fibers are slowly but continually broken down and renewed.

Smooth muscle cells occur as circular sleeves surrounding the bronchi and bronchioles. They dilate when the body needs large volumes of air, for example, during exercise. When these muscles contract, as on exposure to irritant gases, they make the conducting airways narrower, increasing resistance to air flow. Smooth muscle cells also surround blood vessels that enter the lung. They control the distribution of blood flow to specific alveoli and determine how hard the right side of the heart must work to pump blood through the pulmonary blood vessels.

Defense Mechanisms

The respiratory system has elaborate defense mechanisms against damage from exposure to potentially hazardous particles and gases (table 2-1). Particles of 1-2 micrometers are the optimal size for reaching the alveoli. Relatively large particles get trapped in nasal hairs and never enter the lower respiratory tract, or they are removed by coughing or sneezing. Somewhat smaller particles (down to about 2 micrometers) enter the trachea but land on the airway surfaces and stick to the surface mucus. The finest particles settle less efficiently and are usually exhaled (19).

In the alveoli, some material may dissolve and be absorbed into the bloodstream or interstitial fluid. Particles that do not dissolve may be phagocytized by macrophages and the phagocytic cells are either swept up the tracheobronchial tree on the mucous blanket or they migrate to the interstitial fluid. Some insoluble particles may remain sequestered in the lung.

The immune system also plays an important role in protecting the lungs. A detailed description is beyond the scope of this background paper, but OTA has previously addressed immune system responses to toxic substances (23). Briefly, exposure to many substances, particularly those containing protein of animal or vegetable origin, sensitizes cells of the immune system. The cells respond with a complex variety of reactions to destroy or immobilize the inhaled substance. These processes, however, are often accompanied by inflammation of the surrounding tissues, which is part of the repair process necessary to restore normal function. Repeated exposure and inflammation is thought to result in serious and permanent tissue damage.

RESPIRATORY RESPONSE TO HARMFUL SUBSTANCES

When defenses are overcome or an agent is particularly toxic, the respiratory system can be injured. Damage occurs when defense and repair mechanisms cannot keep pace with damage wrought by acute exposures to relatively large amounts of harmful substances or by chronic exposures to small amounts of harmful substances. Some damage may result from the repair process itself. Some of the most common and best understood conditions are described here, excluding cancer, which is not being considered in this background paper.

Chronic Bronchitis

People with chronic bronchitis have increased numbers of secretory cells in the bronchial tree. They produce an excess of mucus and have a recurrent or chronic cough, familiar to many as "smoker's cough." This excess secretion of mucus may lead to impairment of normal clearance mechanisms. The normal ciliary movement cannot cope with this large volume of mucus, and consequently, it takes longer for particles to

Table 2-1—Respiratory Tract Clearance Mechanisms

Upper respiratory tract	Tracheobronchial tree	Pulmonary region
Mucociliary transport	Mucociliary transport	Macrophage transport
Sneezing	Coughing	Interstitial pathways
Nose wiping and blowing	Dissolution (for soluble particles)	Dissolution (for soluble and "insoluble" particles)
Dissolution (for soluble particles)		

SOURCE: R.B. Schlesinger, "Biological Disposition of Airborne Particles: Basic Principles and Application to Vehicular Emissions," *Air Pollution, the Automobile, and Public Health,* A.Y. Watson (ed.) (Washington, DC: National Academy Press, 1988).

be removed from the lungs of patients with chronic bronchitis than it does in healthy people. This reduced clearance makes people with chronic bronchitis more susceptible to respiratory infections because bacteria entering the respiratory tract are not removed efficiently.

Almost 12 million people in the United States suffer from chronic bronchitis (1). The epidemiologic evidence linking smoking and chronic bronchitis is overwhelming (10,24). Epidemiologic studies have also shown a correlation between chronic bronchitis and exposure to industrial dust (5,15). In addition, recurrent infections may play a role in the development of chronic bronchitis (4,6). In industrialized urban areas, periods of heavy pollution with sulfur dioxide and particulates have shown a correlation with increased symptoms of chronic bronchitis or mortality due to chronic bronchitis (13,21,22,27).

Emphysema

The lung is supported by a network of protein fibers made of collagen and elastin. In people with emphysema, some of these fibers are lost and the structural network is disrupted. The fiber network in the damaged area becomes rearranged, resulting in destruction of the walls of the alveoli. The air spaces become enlarged, and part of the surface area available for gas exchange is lost (figure 2-6). Less force is needed to

Figure 2-6—Effects of Emphysema on Alveolar Walls

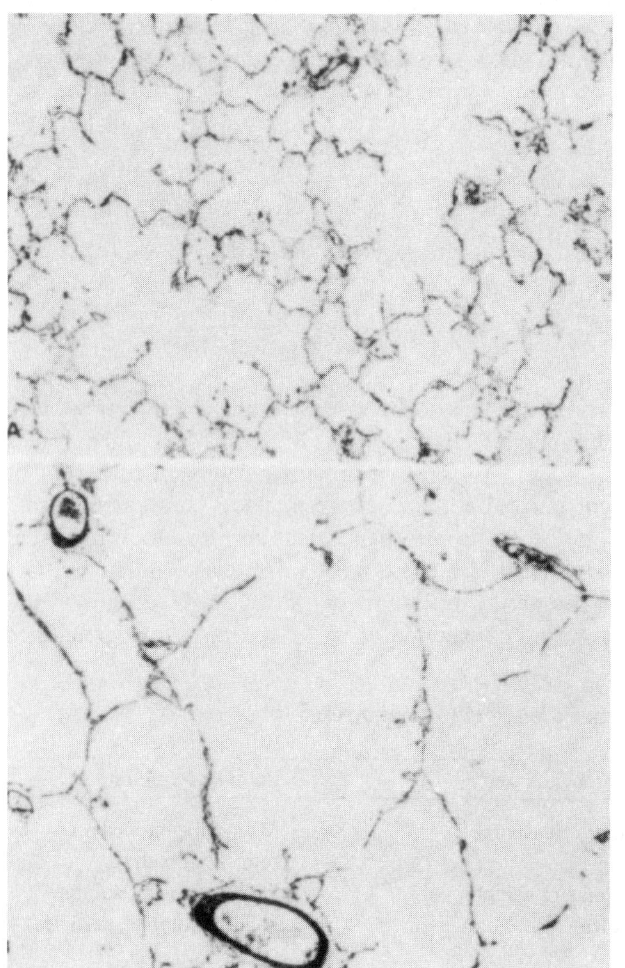
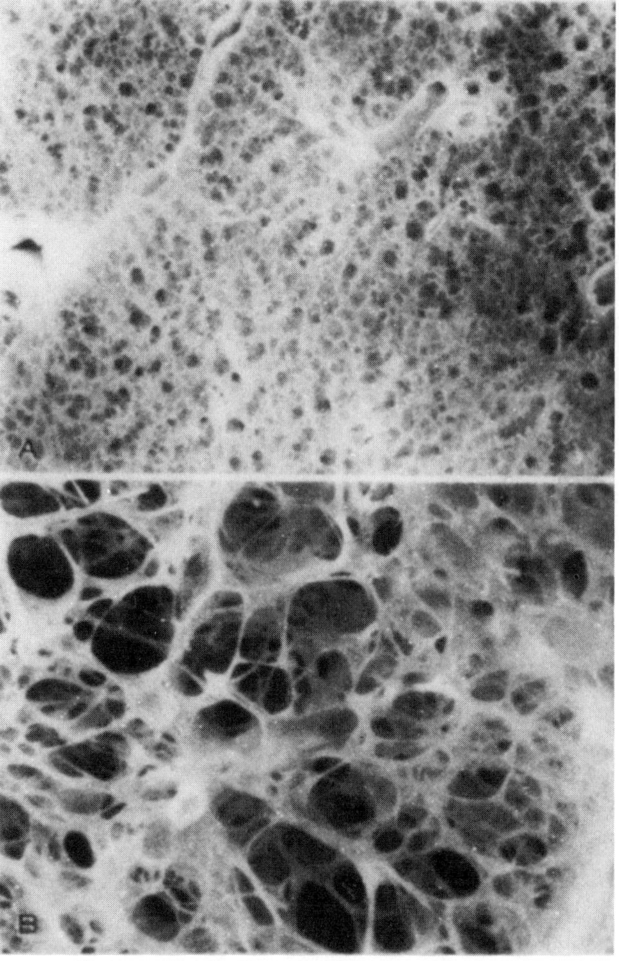

Photo credit : D. Costa, Environmental Protection Agency

The top photo in each column shows normal lung tissue while the bottom photos show destruction
of the walls of the alveoli due to emphysema.

expand the lung, but air may remain trapped in the lung during exhalation because its ability to recoil is impaired.

Nearly 2 million Americans, mostly adults over age 45, have emphysema (1). Emphysema usually develops gradually. Impairment progresses steadily and includes labored breathing and wheezing. It frequently occurs along with chronic bronchitis. [1]

There is a strong correlation between emphysema and heavy cigarette smoking (2). Industrial exposure to cadmium is also associated with emphysema (8). Some people have a genetic predisposition to the development of emphysema. In particular, people who have an inherited deficiency in the amount of a serum protein called alpha$_1$-antitrypsin are more likely to develop emphysema (14,31), especially if they smoke.

Byssinosis

Textile workers exposed to cotton, hemp, flax, and sisal dusts for several years may develop acute symptoms, such as chest tightness, wheezing, and cough. After long-term exposure, they may develop chronic symptoms of respiratory disease indistinguishable from chronic bronchitis but called byssinosis. Bronchoconstriction in this disease is not the result of an allergic response. It is apparently caused by a substance ("a histamine releasing agent") found, for example, in cotton seeds that are present as contaminants in raw cotton fiber.

Asthma

Asthma is a chronic disease of the airways in which symptoms appear intermittently. In healthy people, the smooth muscle surrounding the airways responds to strong environmental stimuli by contracting, increas-

ing the resistance to airflow. Patients with asthma develop more intense constriction of the smooth muscle in response to milder stimuli than do healthy people. The reasons for this response are unclear. Inflammation is usually present, and is thought to play a key role in the disease. In addition to bronchial hyper-responsiveness, people with asthma have intermittent symptoms of wheezing, chest tightening, or cough.

The disease varies from individual to individual not only in its severity, but in the types of agents that provoke an attack. Some people develop symptoms

Table 2-2—Causes of Occupational Asthma

Complex salts of platinum
    Ammonium hexachloroplatinate
Isocyanates
    Toluene di-isocyanate; hexamethylene di-isocyanate;
        naphthalene di-isocyanate
Epoxy resin curing agents
    Phthalic acid anhydride; trimellitic acid anyhydride;
        triethylene tetramine
Colophony fumes
Proteolytic enzymes
    Bacillus subtilis (alkalase)
Laboratory animal urine
    Rats, mice, guinea pigs, rabbits, locusts
Flour and grain dusts
    Barley, oats, rye, wheat
Formaldehyde
Antibiotics
    Penicillin
Wood dusts
    South African boxwood (*Gonioma kamassi*):
        Canadian red cedar
        (*Thuja plicata*); Mansonia (*Sterculiacea altissima*)
Natural gums
    Gum acacia, gum arabic, tragacanth

SOURCE: D.J. Weatherall, J.G.G. Ledingham, and D.A. Warrell (eds.), Oxford Textbook of Medicine (New York, NY: Oxford University Press, 1987).

---

1 Emphysema and chronic bronchitis are two distinct processes. Emphysema, however, can only be diagnosed definitively after death, by direct examination of lung tissue. Incidence data are derived from postmortem surveys. These surveys show that almost all adult lungs have some signs of emphysema, although only a minority of adults have symptoms or disability. Clinicians and epidemiologists dealing with the living use the synonomous terms chronic obstructive pulmonary disease (COPD), chronic obstructive airway disease (COAD), and chronic obstructive lung disease (COLD) to describe patients whose airflow is limited as a result of bronchitis, emphysema, or a combination of the two.

only in response to one stimulus. In the United States, for example, many people with asthma develop symptoms only during the ragweed pollen season in late summer. Others have clear responses to particular occupational agents (table 2-2). But other patients respond to many substances. Even the mechanisms of the disease vary among individuals. In some people with asthma, the response seems to occur through an immunologic reaction, but in other people, the immune system does not seem to be involved in the response. Other mechanisms are the subject of active research. It may be that asthma is a family of diseases with similar symptoms but different underlying causes and mechanisms.

In the United States, about 11.5 million people have asthma (1). Children, African-Americans, and inner city residents are affected disproportionately (11). Both the prevalence and the severity of asthma in the United States have been increasing in recent years (12,30).

Although its causes are not precisely known, over 200 substances have been identified that can induce symptoms (16). In addition, attacks can be provoked by exercise, cold air, airway drying, infections, and emotional upsets. Sulfur dioxide, a component of air pollution, causes severe narrowing of asthmatic airways at concentrations as low as 0.5 parts per million (3,20). Exposure to respirable particles has been associated with reduced lung function and increased symptoms in asthmatic children (18), increased hospital visits (17) and increased rates of acute bronchitis, particularly in asthmatic children (9).

Pulmonary Fibrosis

Pulmonary fibrosis is a family of related disorders characterized by scar tissue in the lungs. Chronic injury and inflammation can result in the formation of scar tissue in the lung, similar to the process of normal wound-healing. In pulmonary fibrosis, however, the wounding and formation of scar tissue is not a specific event in a specific location. Rather it can be a chronic, continuing process that involves the entire lung or there may be scattered, nonuniform scarring. People with pulmonary fibrosis must work harder to breathe, have poor gas exchange, and often have a dry cough.

The inflammatory response of the lung varies depending on the substance causing the injury. In many cases, causative agents are clearly established. Pulmonary fibrosis is known to be caused by exposure to high concentrations of silica, asbestos, and other dusts (table 2-3).

Extrinsic Allergic Alveolitis

Workers sometimes develop severe immune responses to substances in the workplace, particularly to inhaled plant and animal dusts. The disease is easy to recognize in its acute form because workers themselves quickly learn to associate the flu-like symptoms with dust exposure. The chronic form, which seems to occur in response to low-level chronic exposures to dusts rather than high-level exposures, is more insidious. The chronic form of the disease usually progresses very slowly, but can result in pulmonary fibrosis.

Many causative agents have been identified. Most are molds or fungi contaminating organic material, or they are proteins found in animal or bird droppings. The best known form is probably farmers' lung, which is caused by allergies to *Micropolyspora faeni*, found in moldy hay, straw, and grain. There are many other examples, however, including bird fanciers' lung, associated with proteins found in parakeet and pigeon droppings; dog house disease, associated with a mold found in straw dog bedding; paprika splitters' lung, associated with a mold found in paprika; and maple bark strippers' lung, also associated with a mold.

LUNG DISEASE AND EXPOSURE TO TOXIC SUBSTANCES

The Federal Government, as described further in chapter 4, funds research in pulmonary diseases. Some research is aimed at understanding the mechanisms by which a particular substance damages the respiratory system. Often, this knowledge can provide insight into the mechanisms by which other toxic substances cause damage. Many toxic substances cause similar reactions in the respiratory system simply because the respiratory system has a limited range of responses to insults. Asthmatic attacks, for example, are induced by a wide variety of substances, and, similarly, many substances cause pulmonary fibrosis. Careful study of the effect of

Table 2-3—Industrial Toxicants Producing Lung Disease

Toxicant	Common name of disease	Occupational source	Chronic effect	Acute effect
Asbestos	Asbestosis	Mining, construction, shipbuilding, manufacture of asbestos-containing material		Fibrosis, pleural calcification, lung cancer, pleural mesothelioma
Aluminum dust	Aluminosis	Manufacture of aluminum products, fireworks, ceramics, paints, electrical goods, abrasives	Cough, shortness of breath	Interstitial fibrosis
Aluminum abrasives	Shaver's disease, corundum smelter's lung, bauxite lung	Manufacture of abrasives, smelting	Alveolar edema	Interstitial fibrosis, emphysema
Ammonia		Ammonia production, manufacture of fertilizers, chemical production, explosives	Upper and lower respiratory tract irritation, edema	Chronic bronchitis
Arsenic		Manufacture of pesticides, pigments, glass alloys	Bronchitis	Lung cancer, bronchitis, laryngitis
Beryllium	Berylliosis	Ore extraction, manufacture of alloys, ceramics	Severe pulmonary edema, pneumonia	Fibrosis, progressive dyspnea, interstitial granulomatosis, cor pulmonale
Cadmium oxide		Welding, manufacture of electrical equipment, alloys, pigments, smelting	Cough, pneumonia	Emphysema, cor pulmonale
Carbides of tungsten, titanium, tantalum	Hard metal disease	Manufacture of cutting edges on tools	Hyperplasia and metaplasia of bronchial epithelium	Peribronchical and perivascular fibrosis
Chlorine		Manufacture of pulp and paper, plastics, chlorinated chemicals	Cough, hemoptysis, dyspnea, tracheobronchitis, bronchopneumonia	
Chromium (VI)		Production of Cr compounds, paint pigments, reduction of chromite ore	Nasal irritation, bronchitis	Lung cancer fibrosis
Coal dust	Pneumoconiosis	Coal mining		Fibrosis
Cotton dust	Byssinosis	Manufacture of textiles	Chest tightness, wheezing, dyspnea	Reduced pulmonary function, chronic bronchitis
Hydrogen fluoride		Manufacture of chemicals, photographic film, solvents, plastics	Respiratory irritation, hemorrhagic pulmonary edema	

Table 2-3—Industrial Toxicants Producing Lung Disease (Cont'd)

Toxicant	Common name of disease	Occupational source	Chronic effect	Acute effect
Iron oxides	Siderotic lung disease; silver finisher's lung, hematite miner's lung, arc welder's lung	Welding, foundry work, steel manufacture, hematite mining, jewelry making	Cough	Silver finisher's: subpleural and perivascular aggregations of macrophages; hematite miner's: diffuse fibrosis-like pneumonconiosis; arc welder's; bronchitis
Isocyanates		Manufacture of plastics, chemical industry	Airway irritation, cough, dyspnea	Asthma, reduced pulmonary function
Kaolin	Kaolinosis	Pottery making		Fibrosis
Manganese	Manganese pneumonia	Chemical and metal industries	Acute pneumonia, often fatal	Recurrent pneumonia
Nickel		Nickel ore extraction, smelting, electronic electroplating, fossil fuels,	Pulmonary edema, delayed by 2 days (NiCO)	Squamous cell carcinoma of nasal cavity and lung
Oxides of nitrogen		Welding, silo filling, explosive manufacture	Pulmonary congestion and edema	
Ozone		Welding, bleaching flour, deodorizing	Pulmonary edema	Emphysema
Phosgene		Production of plastics, pesticides, chemicals	Edema	Bronchitis
Perchloroethylene		Dry cleaning, metal degreasing, grain fumigating	Edema	
Silica	Silicosis, pneumoconioisis	Mining, stone cutting, construction, farming, quarrying		Fibrosis
Sulfur dioxide		Manufacture of chemicals, refrigeration, bleaching, fumigation	Bronchoconstriction, cough, chest tightness	
Talc	Talcosis	Rubber industry, cosmetics		Fibrosis
Tin	Stanosis	Mining, processing of tin		Widespread mottling of x-ray without clinical signs
Vanadium		Steel manufacture	Airway irritation and mucus production	Chronic bronchitis

SOURCE: T. Gordon, and M.O. Amdur " Responses of the Respiratory System to Toxic Agents," *Casarett and Doull's Toxocology: The Basic Science of Poisons,* M.O. Amdur, I. Doull and C.D. Klassen, (ed.) (New York, NY: Pergamon Press, 1991).

one substance helps researchers to understand the effects of other substances.

Other research is aimed at identifying which substances cause the development of disease, what levels of exposure are harmful, and why responses to toxicants differ among subgroups of the population (25). Identifying specific causes of respiratory diseases is no simple matter because different substances can cause similar kinds of damage, and, conversely, one substance can cause several kinds of damage. It is easier to establish causal relationships when a defined population exposed to high levels of a particular substance exhibits characteristic symptoms or changes in respiratory function. Dozens of examples among occupational groups illustrate how high-level exposures have allowed identification of many causes of occupational asthma, pulmonary fibrosis, and extrinsic allergic alveolitis (table 2-3).

It is more difficult to determine the effects of substances to which many people are exposed at much lower levels than the heavy occupational exposures. Five major components of air pollution, carbon monoxide, sulfur oxides, hydrocarbons, particulates, and oxidants, are widely distributed in varying concentrations throughout the United States. No single, well-defined group is exposed to any one of these at exceptionally high levels; instead virtually everyone is exposed at some level. Large proportions of the population are also exposed to varying concentrations of common indoor air pollutants such as environmental tobacco smoke; nitrogen oxides (from gas stoves); woodsmoke; allergens of the house dust mite, cats, rodents, and cockroaches; and formaldehyde and other volatile organic compounds. Sorting out particular effects of each of these substances is quite different from identifying the cause of bird fanciers' lung or maple bark strippers' lung. The high background level of respiratory disease in the population at large also makes pinpointing particular causal agents more difficult. The kinds of tests and studies aimed at elucidating the relationships between respiratory diseases and exposure to indoor and outdoor air pollutants are explored in the next chapter.

CHAPTER 2 REFERENCES

1. Adams, P.F., and Benson, V., *Current Estimates From the National Health Interview Survey, 1989,* National Center for Health Statistics, Vital Health Stat. 10(176), 1990.

2. Auerbach, O., Hammond, E.C., Garfinkel, L., et al., "Relation of Smoking and Age to Emphysema: Whole-Lung Section Study," *New England Journal of Medicine* 286:853-857, 1972.

3. Balmes, J.R., Fine, J.M., and Sheppard, D., "Symptomatic Bronchoconstriction After Short-term Inhalation of Sulfur Dioxide," *American Review of Respiratory Disease* 136:1117-1121, 1987.

4. Barker, D.J.P., and Osmond, C., "Childhood Respiratory Infection and Adult Chronic Bronchitis in England and Wales," *British Medical Journal* 293:1271-1275, 1986.

5. Becklake, M.R., "Chronic Airflow Limitation: Its Relationship to Work in Dusty Occupations," *Chest* 88:608-17, 1985.

6. Colley, J.R.T., Douglas, J.W.B., and Reid, D.D., "Respiratory Disease in Young Adults: Influence of Early Childhood Respiratory Tract Illness, Social Class, Air Pollution and Smoking," *British Medical Journal* 3:195-198, 1973.

7. Crystal, R.G., West, J.B., Barnes, P.J., et al., (eds.), *The Lung: Scientific Foundations* (New York NY: Raven Press, 1991).

8. Davison, A.G., Newman Taylor, A.J., Darbyshire, J., et al., "Cadmium Fume Inhalation and Emphysema," *The Lancet* Mar. 26, 1988, pp. 663-667.

9. Dockery, D.W., Speizer, F.E., Stram, D.O., et al., "Effects of Inhalable Particles on Respiratory Health of Children," *American Review of Respiratory Disease* 139(3):587-594, March 1989.

10. Doll, R., and Peto, R., "Mortality in Relation to Smoking: 20 Years' Observations on Male British Doctors," *British Medical Journal* 2:1525-1536, 1976.

11. Evans, R., Mullally, D.I., Wilson, R.W., et al., "National Trends in the Morbidity and Mortality of Asthma in the U.S.," *Chest* 91(suppl. 6):65S-74S, 1987.

12. Gergen, P.J., and Weiss, K.B., "Changing Patterns of Asthma Hospitalization Among Children: 1979-1987," *Journal of the American Medical Association* 264:1688-1692, 1990.

13. Gordon, T., and Amdur, M.O. "Responses of the Respiratory System to Toxic Agents," *Casarett and Doull's Toxicology: The Basic Science of Poisons* M.O. Amdur et al. (eds.) (New York, NY: Pergamon Press, 1991).

14. Mittman, C., "Summary of Symposium of Pulmonary Emphysema and Proteolysis," *American Review of Respiratory Disease* 105:430-448, 1972.

15. Morgan, W.K.C., "Industrial Bronchitis," *British Journal of Industrial Medicine* 35:285-91, 1978.

16. Newman Taylor, A.J., "Occupational Asthma," *Thorax* 35:241-245, 1980.

17. Pope, C.A., III, "Respiratory Hospital Admissions Associated With PM$_{10}$ Pollution in Utah, Salt Lake, and Cache Valleys," *Archives of Environmental Health* 46(2):90-97, March/April 1991.

18. Pope, C.A. III, Dockery, D.W., Spengler, J.D., et al., "Respiratory Health and PM$_{10}$ Pollution: A Daily Time Series Analysis," *American Review of Respiratory Disease* 144(3 Pt. 1):668-674, 1991.

19. Schlesinger, R.B., "Biological Disposition of Airborne Particles: Basic Principles and Application to Vehicular Emissions," *Air Pollution, the Automobile, and Public Health,* A.Y. Watson, et al. (eds.) (Washington, DC: National Academy Press, 1988).

20. Sheppard, D., Saisho, A., Nadel, J.A., et al., "Exercise Increases Sulfur Dioxide-Induced Bronchoconstriction in Asthmatic Subjects," *American Review of Respiratory Disease* 123:486-491, 1981.

21. Sherrill, D.L., Lebowitz, and Burrows, B., "Epidemiology of Chronic Obstructive Pulmonary Disease," *Clinics in Chest Medicine* 11:375-387, 1990.

22. Speizer, F., "Studies of Acid Aerosols in Six Cities and in a New Multi-city Investigation: Design Issues," *Environmental Health Perspectives* 79:61-68, 1989.

23. U.S. Congress, Office of Technology Assessment, *Identifying and Controlling Immunotoxic Substances-Background Paper,* OTA-BP-BA-75 (Washington, DC: U.S. Government Printing Office, April 1991).

24. U.S. Department of Health and Human Services, *The Health Consequences of Smoking. Chronic Obstructive Airways Disease: A Report of the Surgeon General,* U.S. Department of Health and Human Services, Public Health Service, Office on Smoking and Health, 1984.

25. Utell, M.J., and Frank, R. (eds.), *Susceptibility to Inhaled Pollutants, ASTM STP 1024,* (Philadelphia, PA: American Society for Testing and Materials, 1989).

26. Utell, M.J., and Samet, J.M., "Environmentally Mediated Disorders of the Respiratory Tract," *Medical Clinics of North America* 74(2):291-306, 1990.

27. Waller, R.E., "Atmospheric Pollution," *Chest* 96(3):363S-368S, 1989.

28. Weatherall, D.J., Ledingham, J.G.G., and Warrell, D.A. (eds.), *Oxford Textbook of Medicine* (New York, NY: Oxford University Press, 1987).

29. Weibel, E.R., *The Pathway for Oxygen: Structure and Function in the Mammalian Respiratory System* (Cambridge, MA: Harvard University Press, 1984).

30. Weiss, K.B., and Wagener, D.K., "Changing Patterns of Asthma Mortality," *Journal of the American Medical Association* 264:1683-1687, 1990.

31. Welch, M.H., Guenter, C.A., Hammersten, J.F., "Precocious Emphysema and alpha$_1$-Antitrypsin Deficiency," *Advances in Internal Medicine* 17:379-92, 1971.

Pulmonary Toxicology and Epidemiology

Pulmonary Toxicology and Epidemiology

INTRODUCTION

As individuals move from home to work to various outdoor environments, they breathe air of divergent composition and quality. In addition to the oxygen needed for survival, people inhale a "soup" of gases and particles. The ingredients of that soup range from benign to lethal in their potential and actual effects on the human lung.

Obvious health concerns in the outdoor air include particulate matter, sulfur oxides, nitrogen oxides, ozone, and carbon monoxide—those pollutants associated with a heavily industrialized, fossil-fuel based economy. Workplace concerns differ greatly among occupations, but typically include organic and inorganic dusts and the vapors from various chemicals. Concerns also focus on "indoor" (e.g., home, school, office) air, where substances as ubiquitous as formaldehyde, tobacco smoke, asbestos, woodsmoke, and molds stand accused as potential contributors to respiratory disease.

Exposure to airborne toxicants varies considerably among individuals and among populations. A taxi driver who cooks over a gas stove receives a regulated (vehicle emissions) and unregulated (stove emissions) dose of nitrogen dioxide, while a homemaker in an all-electric home may receive a wholly unregulated dose of formaldehyde (offgassing from furnishings or insulation). A school-age child of smoking parents may be exposed to air pollutants subject to legislative controls (e.g., asbestos in schools) and uncontrolled pollutants (e.g., tobacco smoke in the home) with known synergistic effects. Residents downwind of a coal-burning power plant may worry about sulfur dioxide and particulate matter, while the miners who supply the fuel may worry more about coal dust. Policymakers and regulators must determine how best to protect human health from the potential ill effects of these multiple exposures to toxicants. They wrestle with technical questions (e.g., is there solid evidence that Substance

X causes human health problems? If so, at what concentrations?) and socio-economic questions (e.g., does the benefit of avoiding a particular health problem outweigh the cost of reducing the toxic exposure that causes it?).

This chapter examines how toxicology and epidemiology contribute to decisions on whether or how to regulate substances because of pulmonary toxicity (box 3-A). The chapter first describes the framework for most regulatory decision making—risk assessment—and then describes the types of technologies available to complete each step of that process with regard to inhaled pulmonary toxicants. The technologies covered include those that enable assessment of exposure and dose and assessment of health effects. Finally, this chapter examines whether remaining questions about the noncancer health risks of pulmonary toxicants merely await application of existing technologies or whether answers will require development of new tools.

FRAMEWORK FOR STUDYING TOXICANTS

Early efforts to identify and control pulmonary toxicants in the United States were directed at substances that induced obvious disease in highly exposed individuals. In recent years efforts have focused more on attempts to protect the general population from the more nebulous "unacceptable risk of disease" at much lower exposure levels (34). But the objective of reducing mortality and morbidity remains. The statutes that authorize control of pollutants to protect human health explicitly or implicitly require a substantial amount of proof that a substance causes disease or injury before the substance can be subjected to regulatory controls. The framework in which such proof is sought is generally referred to as risk assessment.

Risk assessment is the process of characterizing and quantifying potential adverse health effects that

---

Box 3-A—General Principles of Toxicology

To evaluate the toxic nature of a substance, including its pulmonary toxicity, scientists have developed several general criteria for consideration, including:

Nature of the Toxic Substance. Toxicologists try to determine the characteristics that render a chemical toxic. Individual molecules may not be toxic in their native states but become toxic after being metabolized. The size and shape of particles may affect their toxicity.

Dose and Length of Exposure. These parameters, together with rates of metabolism and excretion, determine what quantity of a substance is actually affecting the body. A given substance may be toxic in high doses but nontoxic under conditions of chronic low-dose exposure.

Route of Exposure. The pathway by which a toxicant enters the body (e.g., skin, eye, lungs, or gastrointestinal tract) affects its toxicity. The amount of absorption, ability of the toxicant to combine with native molecules at the entry point (e.g., heavy metals with skin collagen), vulnerability of sensitive areas (e.g., lining of the lung), and condition of the organ at time of contact (e.g., pH and content of the stomach) all play a role in subsequent toxicity. This study examines inhalation exposures.

Species Affected. Toxicants exhibit different levels and effects of toxicity depending on the species on which it is tested.

Age. Susceptibility to a toxicant varies with age—the young and the old generally being the most susceptible.

State of Health. The health status of an individual, including the presence of disease, can greatly affect toxicity response. For example, people with asthma may suffer adverse effects from substances that do no harm to most individuals.

Individual Susceptibility. Host factors such as genetic predisposition affect the response of an individual to a toxicant.

Presence of Other Agents. Toxicology often involves evaluating one substance in isolation, yet the body is seldom exposed to agents in this manner. Knowledge about toxic effects of multiple substances is not well-developed because of the practical limitations of testing the infinite number of combinations.

Adaptation/Tolerance. Biological adaptation to a toxicant often occurs when chronically low doses are presented. Adaptation/tolerance must be factored into evaluating the range of individual responsiveness to a toxicant.

SOURCE: Office of Technology Assessment, 1992, based on M.A. Ottoboni, *The Dose Makes the Poison* (Berkeley, CA: Vincente Books, 1984).

---

may result from exposures to harmful physical or chemical agents in the environment. As practiced in U.S. Federal agencies, it generally involves four essential elements:

- hazard identification;
- dose-response assessment;
- exposure assessment; and
- risk characterization (9,27).

The process of *hazard identification* attempts to determine whether a particular substance or mixture of substances can create a measurable health effect. *Dose-response assessment* identifies the health effects caused by a given dose of the substance under study. *Exposure assessment* applies measurement and extrapolation technologies to determine what level of human exposure can be anticipated. *Risk characterization* integrates the results of the first three steps to estimate the incidence of a health effect for a given population under various conditions of human exposure (24,27).

Bringing a risk assessment of a suspected pulmonary toxicant to a satisfactory conclusion poses tricky problems for an investigator. Hazard identification may involve laboratory and field studies. In vitro tests at the cellular level may indicate that a substance causes a biological response but fail to address whether the effect would be adverse in the whole animal, where defense mechanisms may prevent the toxicant from reaching the cells being tested. Dose-response assessments often are performed on animals rather than humans (particularly when new substances are being studied), which requires knowledge of whether animals and humans would respond similarly to the substance under study. Animal tests of acute exposures can be conducted with relative ease, but tests of low-level, chronic exposures are time-consuming and costly. Lack of emissions data, lack of knowledge about how substances are transported in the air, and lack of adequate monitoring devices typically complicate the exposure assessment. The following sections on Exposure Assessment and Dosimetry and on Health Effects Assessment describe technologies available for risk assessment of pulmonary toxicants and limits of those technologies.

EXPOSURE ASSESSMENT AND DOSIMETRY

Exposure to a contaminant has been defined as contact between a person and a physical or chemical agent. Exposure differs from *biologically effective dose,* which is the amount of a contaminant that interacts with cells and results in altered physiologic function. Regulators direct their efforts toward controlling exposures to populations that can reasonably be expected to result in harmful, biologically effective doses to individuals within those populations. The technologies of exposure assessment and dosimetry contribute to these efforts.

Exposure assessment is the estimation of the magnitude, frequency, duration, and route of exposure to a substance with the potential to cause adverse health effects. *Dosimetry* is the estimation of the amount of a toxicant that reaches the target site, in this case the lung, following exposure (30). The following subsections first describe devices that can be used to estimate exposure and determine the amount of a toxicant actually retained by the lung, and then describe technologies available to help scientists predict the biologically effective dose that will be produced by a given human exposure (figure 3-1).

Estimating Exposure and Biologically Effective Dose

A series or combination of physical and biological events may affect whether a toxicant that becomes airborne will create a health effect. Toxicants may be transported and transformed in the environment before human contact. Defense mechanisms in the respi-

ratory system may remove or transform a toxicant before it causes damage. This section describes technologies to measure actual and potential exposures to toxicants and technologies to measure retention by the lung.

Exposure

Exposure to airborne toxic substances traditionally has been estimated by sampling community and workplace air. Continuous samplers, used to measure gases, and integrating samplers, used to measure particles, are placed at one or more fixed sites in urban and nonurban areas (22). Contaminant concentrations derived from such measurements of the outdoor air have often been used to estimate an individual's average acute or lifetime exposure. Such estimates assume that all contact with pollutants occurs in the outdoors and that the breathing zone concentration is identical to that at fixed-site monitors.

In reality, people come into contact with polluted air in many different environments. Sophisticated monitoring devices now permit consideration of the multiple opportunities for people to come into contact with polluted air. Indirect (microenvironmental) and direct (personal) monitoring, combined with outdoor measurements, help scientists arrive at more accurate estimates of individuals' total exposure to airborne pollutants. Indirect monitoring uses traditional air sampling techniques but applies them to microenvironments—various indoor (e.g., homes, commercial buildings, worksites, vehicles) and outdoor (e.g., highways, industrial sites, backyards) sites. Personal monitoring requires individuals to wear or carry a sampling device throughout the study period and, generally, to log their daily activities to help associate measured exposures with their sources. Studies have demonstrated the effectiveness of personal monitoring devices (45), but scientists generally agree that detection limits and reliability need improvement. Techniques to enhance or supplement personal activity logs, such as personal location monitors, would also increase the precision achievable with personal monitoring devices (22).

Biologically Effective Dose

Several factors influence the amount of an inhaled contaminant that actually reaches lung tissues and cells following exposure. An individual at rest inhales less air than an exercising individual because exercise increases the ventilation rate. The ambient exposure can

Figure 3-1—Framework for Exposure Assessment

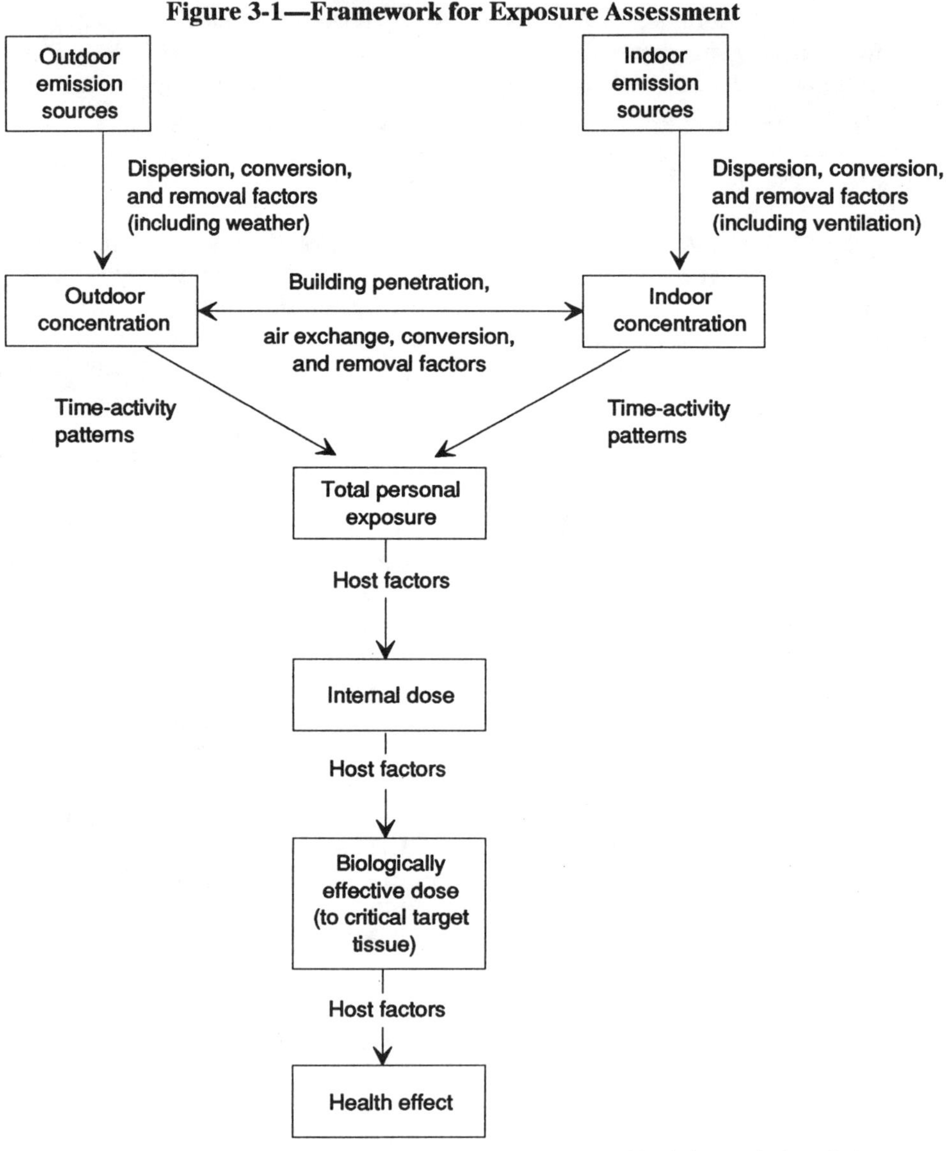

SOURCE: National Research Council, Committee on Epidemiology of Air Pollutants, *Epidemiology and Air Pollution* (Washington, DC: National Academy Press, 1985).

be the same for each, but exercise increases the biologically effective dose. Inhaled toxicants may be removed from the inspired air before they reach the tracheo-bronchial and pulmonary regions (the predominant sites of injury that may lead to changes in pulmonary performance; see ch. 2). But individuals who breathe through their mouths rather than noses (e.g., asthmatics) may lose the benefit of that respiratory defense mechanism. Techniques ranging from measurements of exhaled air to examination of excised lung samples can be used to estimate how much of a substance reaches and is retained by various regions of the lung.

Analysis of exhaled air—Gas chromatography/mass spectroscopy can be used to measure exhaled air for contaminants that were absorbed by the lung. Breath measurements have been shown to correlate with preceding exposures for selected volatile organic compounds (45).

Analysis of body fluids—Sputum and fluid obtained by nasal lavage can be analyzed for the presence of toxic substances. Blood and urine can be analyzed for the presence of toxicants, but current measurements of these fluids generally yield very little or no information about the delivered dose of a toxicant to the lung.

Analysis of the whole lung—Invasive and relatively noninvasive techniques can be used to determine the quantity of particles in the lungs of living subjects. Whole-lung scanning for particles labeled with radioactive tags (performed on an experimental basis) permits determination of the total concentration in the lung of certain types of inhaled particles and the size of the particles. Open-lung biopsy (an invasive technique requiring strong justification in humans) permits direct counting of particles or determination of fiber burden per gram of lung tissue (29). A noninvasive technique, magnetopneumography (MPG), provides a means of actively monitoring the dust retained in the lungs of people exposed to magnetic or magnetizable dusts. MPG can be used intermittently, for test purposes only, or to monitor individuals (particularly workers) for unacceptable rates of dust accumulation. Only magnetic or magnetizable dusts (e.g., asbestos, coal) can be monitored with MPG.

Analysis of samples of lung tissue—Scanning electron microscopy has been used to determine the deposition site, in rat, mouse, and hamster lungs, of particles small enough to reach the conducting airways. It also has permitted quantification of the particles present at selected deposition sites. Transmission electron microscopy has been used to locate inorganic particles in lung tissue, which can then be analyzed to identify the particle type. The techniques allow determination of the chemical composition and structure of a wide range of particles of varying sizes and elemental composition (31).

Determining Physical Properties of a Toxicant

Determination of the physical properties of a toxicant may allow an investigator to predict how a gas or particle will behave in the environment (how it will be dispersed following emission) and in the lung (how it will be deposited and cleared from the respiratory system). This background paper does not address methods for determining atmospheric dispersion but is concerned with methods for determining regional deposition within the lung.

Toxicants are inhaled as *gases, vapors*, or *aerosols* (table 3-1). Many factors influence deposition of gases and aerosols in the lung. For instance, exercise-induced oral (as opposed to nasal) breathing increases the amount of gas or particles that bypasses the nasopharyngeal region and reaches the deep airways. Doses of toxicants that overwhelm normal lung defenses (see ch. 2) can also affect the deposition of gases and particles. The most influential factors in deposition are the physical properties of the substances under study (and the species in which they are tested.

As a general rule, water soluble gases inhaled through the nose will be partially extracted in the upper airways. Less soluble gases will reach the small airways and alveoli. Particle size generally determines the region of the lung affected by particles. Particles with an

Table 3-1—Defining Gases and Aerosols

Gases	Substances that are in the gaseous state at room temperature and pressure.
Vapors	The gaseous phase of a material that is ordinarily a solid or liquid at room temperature and pressure.
Aerosols	Relatively stable suspensions of solid particles or liquid droplets in air.
Dusts	Solid particles formed by grinding, milling, or blasting.
Fumes	Vaporized material formed by combustion, sublimation, or condensation.
Smoke	Aerosol produced by combustion of organic material.
Mist	Aerosols of liquid droplets formed by condensation of liquid on particulate nuclei in the air or by the uptake of liquid by hygroscopic particles.
Fog	See mist.
Smog	Complex mixture of particles and gases formed in the atmosphere by sunlight's effects on nitrogen oxides and volatile organic compounds.

SOURCE: T. Gordon and M. Amdur, "Responses of the Respiratory System to Toxic Agents," in *Cassarett and Doull s Toxicology: The Basic Science of Poisons, 4th edition* (Elmsford, NY: Pergamon Press, 1991), pp. 383-406.

aerodynamic size greater than 10 micrometers are mostly removed in the upper airways, while smaller particles penetrate deeper. Extremely small or extremely thin particles can cross the alveolar epithelial barrier and cause interstitial lung injury (see ch. 2).

Knowledge of the physical properties of a toxicant, coupled with the resultant knowledge of the probable site of deposition, points an investigator to the likely site and type of toxic injury. Actual behavior often differs from predicted behavior, but differences are generally revealed during the investigation.

Determining Species Differences

Toxicologists often try to predict the human health effects of toxicants by first studying them in animals. Animals provide useful models for studying toxicant exposure, but differences in anatomy, biochemistry, physiology, cell biology, and pathology affect the way species respond to airborne toxicants (8,46). Risk assessments of toxic substances generally depend on experimental data obtained from a variety of species, and it is essential to consider and study species differences before selecting the appropriate animal for study and making judgments about whether an exposure/dose administered to an animal has relevance for human health (23).

Respiratory tract anatomy differs significantly among species. Although most mammals have similar respiratory tract components, the structure of those components—which affects how substances behave in the lung—varies (e.g., humans differ from most other animals in the size and shape of the nasal airways, in the pattern of tracheobronchial tree branching, and in alveolar size). In addition to direct study of differences, computer modeling techniques now permit three-dimensional reconstructions of the lung, based on tissue samples, that improve the ability to extrapolate from test results in animals to likely health effects in humans (25).

Breathing patterns and lung defense mechanisms also affect the fate of toxicants in the lung. For instance, humans often breathe through their noses and their mouths, while some other animals (notably the rodents used in toxicology) can only breathe through their noses. These differences have a major impact on deposition of particles. Also, scientists now know that alveo-

lar clearance mechanisms, which are designed to clean out the lung and prevent the type of damage that derives from prolonged exposure, are much faster in some species than in others.

Relative distribution of lung cell types differs among species, which affects the type of damage toxicants can inflict. Similarly, the mechanism of injury may differ among species and by exposure type (e.g., chronic exposure to beryllium causes an immune reaction in human lungs, but beryllium acts through direct cytotoxicity in rat and human lungs at acute exposure levels (19)). Only certain species can be used to test disease states of interest to scientists. For example, rats are generally the species of choice for pulmonary toxicologists, but toxicologists often use guinea pigs when asthmatic responses are in question because guinea pigs have airways more sensitive to bronchoconstriction than most species, and hence share a similarity with human asthmatics.

No single species makes a perfect physical surrogate for humans in studying the health effects of airborne toxicants. In addition to scientific issues, toxicologists must also consider the availability and expense of different species, especially when the effects of chronic, rather than acute, exposure are being studied. Much has been learned about species differences, and scientists are beginning to account for those differences when extrapolating from effects in animals to humans. Most experts agree, however, that increased interspecies comparisons and studies of the mechanisms of injury would increase the utility of animal tests in the risk assessment process.

Summary of Exposure Assessment and Dosimetry Technologies

Technologies that measure the presence of gases and aerosols in the ambient air and at target sites within the body play an essential role in risk assessment of airborne toxicants. These technologies have evolved rapidly and continue to improve estimates of human exposure to toxic substances. Scientists point to important gaps in the "exposure assessment knowledge base," however (29,35). These include, generally:

- Lack of knowledge about the disposition of inhaled gases, vapors, and extremely small particles within the respiratory tract;

- Lack of knowledge about the disposition of gases and aerosols within the respiratory tracts of sensitive individuals and groups within the population;
- Inadequate knowledge of the species differences that may affect interpretation of test results; **and**
- Lack of a sound basis for extrapolating the effects of exposure from high to low concentrations.

The gaps present no insurmountable barriers to effective risk assessment but will require time and resources to fill.

HEALTH EFFECTS ASSESSMENT

A health effects assessment completes two steps of the risk assessment process: hazard identification, by determining whether a substance causes damage, and dose-response assessment, by determining the damage caused by a specific dose. Health effects assessments utilize controlled exposure conditions, as with laboratory and clinical studies, or uncontrolled exposure conditions, as with epidemiologic studies. Each type of study has advantages and disadvantages. To compensate, scientists try to integrate the results of multiple studies in their conclusions (figure 3-2). For instance, laboratory, clinical, and epidemiologic studies have contributed to the decision-making process on permissible ozone exposure levels. The following subsections describe the types of tests that can help investigators reach conclusions about the pulmonary effects of airborne toxicants.

Figure 3-2—Integrated Approach to Identifying Pulmonary Toxicants

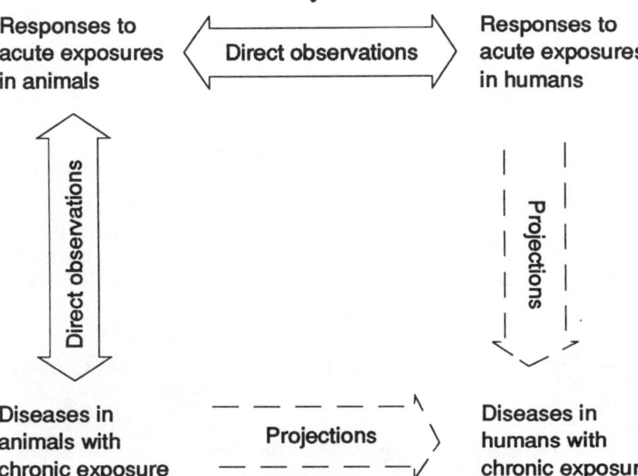

SOURCE: Office of Technology Assessment, 1992, based on M. McClellan, R.O., "Reflections on the Symposium: Susceptibility to Inhaled Pollutants," American Society for Testing and Materials Special Technical Publication 1024, 1989.

Laboratory and Clinical Studies

Laboratory studies and human clinical studies control exposure conditions as closely as possible to limit the influence of extraneous factors on the study. This means, in part, investigators must understand "host factors"—the physical conditions, activity level, and personal habits of the test subject—and other factors, such as time of day or season of the year, that may affect the outcome of a study. It also means investigators choose not only the health effect to study but the amount of toxicant to which tissues and cells, animals, or human volunteers are exposed.

There are drawbacks to studies involving controlled exposure conditions. The fundamental limitation of experiments involving whole animals lies in extrapolating results to humans. As discussed above, techniques are progressing, but scientists are not yet satisfied with their ability to account fcr the differences in human and animal lungs when predicting the effects of a toxicant. In addition, studies using whole animals involve considerable expense and, in some instances, problems with the public's views on animal experimentation. Ethical restraints on human clinical studies—investigators may not inflict harm—place inherent limitations on their use for predicting a toxicant's likelihood of causing a deadly or disabling condition. The intentional simplicity of experiments involving controlled exposures also limits their value for revealing the effects of exposure under "real world" conditions. To isolate the effects of one substance, investigators eliminate other potential toxicants from the air, which may alter the effect the test substance has on the lung.

Technologies to Measure Exposure

Toxicologists performing animal experiments must have the capability to generate the types of chemicals and particles they want to test and the capability to expose the animals to fixed amounts of the test substance(s). Technologies to generate gases and aerosols are well developed (2,26). However, the aerosols generated tend to be far more homogeneous than those encountered in typical urban environments. Exposure occurs in whole-body chambers and in apparatuses permitting head-only and nose-only exposures. Existing systems provide for adequate exposure control and measurement and do not constrain evaluation of test results when system limitations are properly accounted for in the analysis (6). However, continued research is important to understand the implications of the differences in complex, naturally occurring aerosols and those generated for experimental purposes.

Participants in human clinical studies can be exposed to the test substance in exposure chambers (whole-body systems) or through systems using either a facemask, hood, or mouthpiece. Each system has advantages (e.g., exposure chambers permit unencumbered breathing and most accurately simulate normal conditions; mouthpieces are very simple) and disadvantages (e.g., facemasks are difficult to seal; exposure chambers can be expensive to construct and maintain, part of the reason why only four chambers in the United States are effectively operating (37)). It is possible to calibrate the limitations of each system sufficiently to permit adequate evaluation of test results (17). Development of portable exposure chambers could enhance use of that exposure system (37).

Measurements of Effects

Toxicologists can identify pulmonary toxicants through physiologic assays of living subjects, structural analysis of tissues and cells removed from animals or humans, and tests of biochemical responses in removed fluids and cells. The following subsections describe various testing measures.

Physiologic tests—Assays of physiologic function fall into four major categories: measures of ventilatory or gas-exchange functions; measures of increased airway reactivity; measures of particle clearance from the

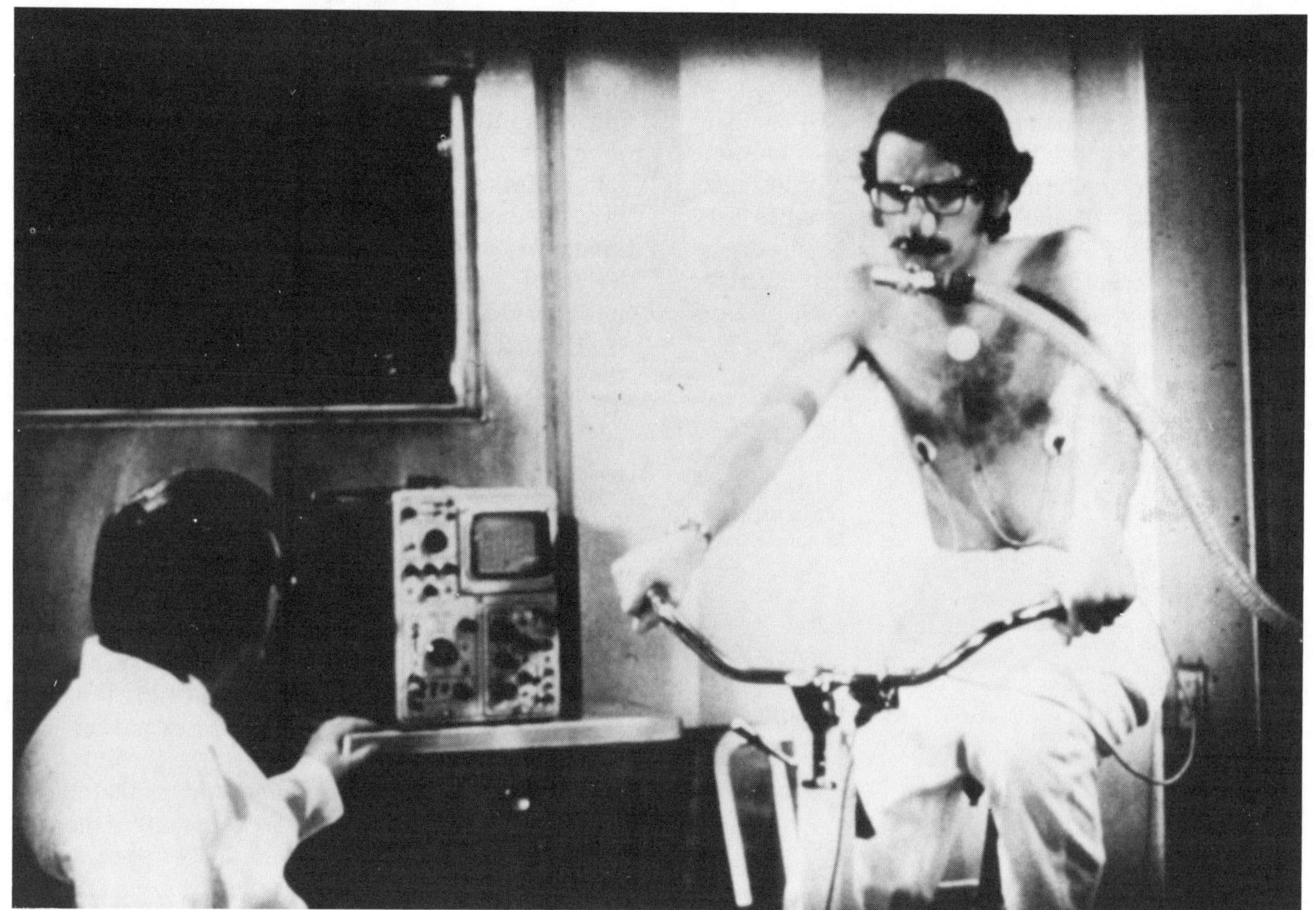

Photo credit: South Coast Air Quality Management District, El Monte, CA

A volunteer undergoes lung function tests while exercising.

lung; and measures of increased permeability of the air-blood barrier. These assays can be used to demonstrate transient and lasting changes in lung function. Functional assays are applied to animals and humans, though specific tests performed vary by species.

Spirometry, which includes various measures of how much and how quickly air can be expelled following a deep breath, constitutes the most common group of respiratory function tests performed in humans. A very frequently used spirometric test measures the amount of air that can be forcibly expelled in 1 second and is referred to as FEV_1 (forced expiratory volume in 1 second). Physicians agree that an FEV_1 below 80 percent of the predicted value (which varies with age, height, and sex) indicates an adverse health effect. EPA has used evidence of decrements in FEV_1 greater than or equal to 10 percent as the basis for regulations. Some studies show that a decrease in FEV_1 following short-term exposure correlates with development of obstructive disease following chronic exposure, but much research remains to be done.

The total amount of air that can be expelled following a deep breath is referred to as forced vital capacity (FVC), and this measure is also a commonly used test. Practitioners of spirometry can chart the air flow rate after 50 percent or 75 percent of the volume has been forcibly expelled (forced expiratory flow of 50 or 75 percent, or FEF_{50} or FEF_{75}). Alternatively, the flow rate between 25 percent and 75 percent of the FVC (maximal midexpiratory flow, or MMEF) can be measured. Some researchers believe that FEF_{50}, FEF_{75}, and MMEF may identify early and subtle damage to airways, which may be the first stage of the type of severe or irreversible damage reflected in the more common measures of FEV_1 or FVC.

Ventilatory function tests that do not require voluntary exhalation maneuvers can be performed in experimental animals. Such tests include measures of the mechanical properties of the lung, i.e., the amount of work required to stretch the lung (inhale) and the work required to push air out of the lung (exhale). Traditional measures of lung mechanics have been used widely in animal studies of toxicants that are pulmonary irritants (7).

The distribution of gases and particles within the lung can also be measured with ventilatory function tests. Single- and multi-breath nitrogen washout tests determine the point in exhalation when the airways begin to close (as evinced by an increase in the nitrogen content of exhaled air). A transient increase in the amount of air left in the lung when the limits of forced exhalation are reached appears to correlate with exposure to pulmonary toxicants. Particle distribution can be examined by measuring the number of particles, administered as an aerosol, in exhaled air and with radioimaging techniques. Efforts are underway to validate such tests, which are not yet in widespread use.

Tests of how well gas diffuses from the lung into the blood system—the diffusing capacity of the lung for carbon monoxide (DL_{CO})—are sometimes included among ventilatory function tests. The tests use carbon monoxide (at harmless dose levels) because it is readily absorbed by the hemoglobin in the blood. The most common DL_{CO} test requires the subject to inhale a mixture of inert gas and carbon monoxide. Changes in the ratio of inert gas to carbon monoxide, as measured in air captured at the end of exhalation, can indicate changes in the lung's diffusing capacity (e.g., if unusually high levels of carbon monoxide remain in the exhaled air, it indicates alterations in the transfer of CO from the lung to the bloodstream).

Measures of airway hyper-reactivity are another type of physiologic test of pulmonary toxicity. These tests assess whether the bronchoconstrictor response to stimuli increases (i.e., whether the airways become hyper-reactive and resist air flow) during or following exposure to inhaled toxicants. In nonspecific airway hyper-reactivity tests, the stimulus for the bronchoconstrictor response may be cold air, exercise, or various pharmacologic agents. This type of testing has proved useful for measuring airway responses to low concentrations of environmental pollutants. In specific airway hyper-reactivity testing, the stimulus is often a common antigen. In nonspecific and specific tests of airway hyper-reactivity, the tests applied following stimulation of the airways involve an airway resistance measurement and a pulmonary function test, usually FEV_1. Airway hyper-reactivity is characteristic of asthma, although it can occur in nonasthmatics. Some researchers suggest airway hyper-reactivity may play an important role in the development of chronic lung diseases.

Particle clearance assessments also provide physiologic evidence of pulmonary toxicity. These assays determine how exposure to toxicants alters the lung's ability to clean itself out. Though several tests are under development, their utility is hindered by the fact that as yet there is no generally accepted range of normal clearance performance. Most tests trace the transport and removal of radiolabeled particles following exposure to a toxicant.

The final, major type of physiologic assay of pulmonary toxicity attempts to measure injury to the air-blood barrier, usually equating injury with increased permeability. Permeability can be determined by measuring ion transport through airway epithelial cells or by measuring the transepithelial transport of molecules into the blood. These tests currently have many drawbacks, and though research appears to be worthwhile, much remains to be done. Permeability of the endothelial cells that line the blood vessels can also be measured, but nondestructive techniques require further validation before they can come into common use.

In 1989, the National Academy of Sciences (NAS) summarized the utility of physiologic assays in identifying pulmonary toxicants (29). A portion of that analysis is reproduced here as table 3-2. The preceding section provides only a cursory overview of the basic types of physiologic tests of pulmonary toxicity, and the reader is referred to the NAS report for detailed descriptions of these and additional tests.

In summary, physiologic function tests provide reasonable measures of response to toxicants but are not particularly specific or sensitive. Changes in function are not unique to individual toxicants (i.e., lung responses to insult are limited). Current tests have limited value in identifying the effects of chronic exposure (which tend to occur insidiously)(44). But when used in tandem with knowledge of exposure, these tests can help identify toxicants.

Structure tests—Injury to lung tissues and cells can, in some instances, be assessed with the naked eye. For instance, in advanced asbestosis the damage asbestos causes to the pleura can be seen unaided in an open chest cavity, and a microscope can provide even greater detail of the damage. Whole lungs or tissues and cells taken from autopsied humans or animals can be directly examined for evidence of toxic effects. X-ray technologies are also useful in structural studies.

Scientists also know that cells of the pulmonary system normally appear in relatively constant numbers and sites within the lung. Examination of tissue from specific regions of the lung can indicate changes in cell populations that are evidence of toxic effects. Mor-

phometry, a technique that employs microscopy to quantify cell populations and structure size using fixed tissue samples, has been widely used to study toxic substances suspected of causing a specific type of injury throughout the lung. Morphometry is more difficult to use to measure toxic effects on small or scattered regions of the lung because tissue samples reflective of the region can be hard to obtain, but improved techniques are under development to assess the gas exchange region of the lung (18). Morphometry can also be used to examine changes in the structure of the pulmonary vasculature. Structural tests may show abnormalities long before changes are detectable by pulmonary function testing. A substantial amount remains to be learned about whether such changes will result in harm, however.

Tests of biochemical and molecular response—Phagocytic pulmonary cells, physiologic mediators, metabolites, enzymes, and other biochemical substances that can be associated with toxic response can be removed from the system by lavage (washing) and the lavage fluid can be analyzed for cellular and biochemical content (20,21). Pulmonary inflammatory responses and immune responses can be measured by examining bronchoalveolar lavage fluid (BALF).

An inflammatory response to a toxic exposure produces enzymes and cells not normally present in BALF. BALF analysis can reveal the degree of inflammation and corresponding stage of any disease process. Aspects of an immune response, such as increased numbers of lymphocytes, can also be measured in BALF. Importantly, immune system cells recovered from BALF can be tested in vitro to determine whether they respond properly to antigen challenge or if they respond to a particular antigen of interest. The functional characteristics of other cell lines obtained from BALF can also be assessed.

Development of safe lavage techniques has contributed immensely to the prospects for pulmonary toxicology. The ability to measure the presence of biochemical substances in BALF has grown faster than knowledge of how those substances correlate to toxicity, but current research is quite promising.

Summary of Technologies Applicable to Laboratory and Clinical Studies

Effective laboratory and clinical studies require technologies to control the dose of a toxicant administered to a test subject and to limit and account for confounding factors. Scientists have developed several exposure technologies and have characterized their potential and drawbacks.

Many established and recently developed technologies exist to measure changes in lung structure and function following exposure to toxic substances. A substantial database exists on the physiological effects of toxicants on animals. Spirometry—as a stand alone measure of ventilatory function and as a component of airway reactivity testing—is the most frequently and easily used technique in human health effects assessments of pulmonary toxicity; additional physiologic measures are under development and may eventually improve the predictive powers of clinical studies of pulmonary toxicity. Microscopy continues to play an important role in laboratory studies, particularly as enhanced by morphometric techniques. The importance of biochemical and molecular measurements, as performed on lavage fluids, is increasing (20,47). Each of these technologies performs well as a diagnostic tool when changes in the lung are gross, but many also measure milder changes that may only represent physiologic variability and, as yet, are not well correlated with changes in pulmonary performance.

Health effects assessments can be performed under acute or chronic exposure conditions. The database on acute exposures is much larger than that on chronic exposures. While this background paper focuses on technologies that identify *whether* a substance causes a toxic effect, it is important to acknowledge that data regarding *how* that effect results in harm should also improve policymakers' ability to deal appropriately with toxic substances.

Epidemiologic Studies

Epidemiology—the study of the distribution and determinants of disease in populations—provides information about the impacts of air pollutants on human populations. It can be used to associate pollutants with disease even before precise mechanisms of cause and effect are understood, although observed associations are often attenuated by serious confounding factors.

Epidemiologic investigations of airborne toxicants share the difficulties inherent in any observational, rather than experimental, studies. For instance, exposure may be hard to assess. Some observers note that knowledge of exposure need not be precise to be mean-

ingful (4), e.g., self-reported exposures to fumes or smoke have correlated well to later measurements, but results based on precise exposure measurements lend themselves more readily to important regulatory decisions. Another problem with epidemiologic studies is that most lung diseases can have more than one cause, and it is difficult to isolate the effects of one airborne substance from another. Finally, it may take studies of quite large populations to reveal small but important effects of airborne toxicants, and such studies can be difficult and costly to undertake. Though hard (sometimes impossible) to conduct, these types of studies can provide evidence of association between exposure and disease that lay and technical people alike find more credible than evidence from laboratory or clinical studies (28).

Epidemiologic studies take many forms. It is possible to study living or deceased populations; diseased populations can be studied for evidence of exposure; healthy populations can be studied for changes in health status following exposure. In all cases, however, some knowledge of exposure and evidence of a defined health effect must be available for results to be meaningful. The following subsections describe the tools available to measure exposure and health effects in epidemiologic studies. Epidemiology uses some of the same technologies as employed in laboratory or clinical studies; some techniques are unique to epidemiology.

Measurements of Exposure

Many of the exposure assessment technologies described previously are applicable to epidemiologic studies. Outdoor, indoor, and personal monitoring devices can be used to provide current exposure information. Records of outdoor measurements collected by public agencies provide historical data of exposure. Population groups can be examined for biological evidence of exposure (e.g., toxic substances found in exhaled air or in autopsied lungs). These measurements typically lack the precision—with regard to exposure to the toxicant under study and to exposure to substances that may alter (confound) the results—obtainable in laboratory and clinical studies, but are used by the scientific community. Moreover, some epidemiologic studies proceed on the basis of self-reported, rather than measured, exposure information.

Measurements of Health Effects

Epidemiologists use many kinds of data to determine health status. Epidemiologic measures include

Table 3-2—Summary of Characteristics of Physiologic Assays

Measure	Characteristics[a] and Ratings[b]					
	A	B	C	D	E	F
Respiratory function						
Spirometry	++	+	++	++	++	+
Lung mechanics						
Dynamic compliance, resistance, and conductance	+	+	++	+	+	+
Oscillation impedance	+-	+	++	++	+-	+-
Static pressure-volume	+	+-	+	+-	+	++
Intrapulmonary distribution						
Single-breath gas washout	+	-	++	+	+	+-
Particle distribution						
Exhaled particles	+-	++	++	++	0	+-
Particle deposition	+-	+	+	+-	0	+-
Alveolar-capillary gas transfer						
CO diffusing capacity	++	+-	++	+-	+-	+
Exercise gas exchange	++	+	++	+	+	+
Airway reactivity						
Nonspecific reactivity	++	+-	++	++	+	+
Specific reactivity	+	+	+	+-	++	++
Particle clearance						
Radiolabeled aerosol	+	+	+-	-	+-	+-
Magnetopneumography	-	-	-	+	0	+-
Air-blood barrier function						
Conducting-airway permeability						
Clearance of inhaled DTPA	+-	+	+	-	0	+-
Transepithelial potential	+-	+	+	+-	0	+-
Alveolar permeability by radiolabeled aerosal	+	+	+	-	+-	+-
Vascular permeability						
Radiolabeled protein leakage	+	+	++	-	0	+
Chest x-ray for edema	++	-	++	+	-	+-
Extravascular lung water by indicator dilution, PET, or NMR	+	+	+	+-	+-	+-
Rebreathing soluble gases	+	+	+	+-	++	+
Endothelial metabolic function	+	+	+	-	+-	+-

some of the same technologies applied in laboratory and clinical studies (e.g., spirometry) and some unique technologies (e.g., questionnaires, historical records). Health effects assessment technologies useful in epidemiologic studies are described briefly below. Box 3-B provides details of a long-term, epidemiologic study of the effects of air pollution on the respiratory health of residents of the Los Angeles area.

Biological tests—Spirometry is often used in epidemiologic studies because it is noninvasive and relatively simple to perform in the field; many

[a]Characteristics:

A. Current State of Development. Considerations in this category included the number of groups using the technique, the availability of the required equipment, the magnitude of the present data base, and the degree of standardization of procedures.

B. Estimated Potential for Development. This category reflected the current estimate of the potential for substantial development of the assay beyond its present state. Although it was recognized that advancements are possible for any assay, this category was intended to reflect potential for substantial technical refinements, adaptation for use in large populations, or advancements in ability to interpret results.

C. Current Applicability of Assay to Humans. Primary considerations were the invasiveness of the technique and the requirement for radionuclides. All the assays can be applied to animals, but some are less suitable than others for evaluating humans.

D. Suitability for Measuring Large Numbers of Subjects. The focus of this category was the suitability of the assay for use in studies of large populations of people, as might be required for evaluating effects of some environmental exposures. Considerations included adaptability of equipment for mobile use, length and nature of subject interaction (i.e., degree of cooperation required), resources required to analyze samples and data, and subject safety. For example, a low rating might suggest a low suitability for field use in evaluating hundreds of subjects of various ages and both sexes, whereas the assay might be quite suitable for studies of dozens of selected subjects brought to a stationary facility.

E. Reproducibility. This category focuses on the variability of results within and between subjects.

F. Interpretability. This category reflects the current understanding of (and degree of consensus as to) pathophysiologic correlates, anatomic sites of effect, and causative agents. For many of the assays, there is little disagreement on the physiologic function affected, but the specific mechanism or site of change is uncertain. For example, it is agreed that reduced carbon monoxide diffusing capacity reflects reduced efficiency of alveolar-capillary gas transfer, but the test does not distinguish among the effects of a thickened membrane, reduced surface area, and reduced capillary blood volume.

[b]Ratings:

0 = Unknown, or information is insufficient.

- = Current information suggests inadequate development, little potential for development, little applicability to humans, poor suitability for large populations, poor reproducibility, or poor interpretability.

+- = Current information suggests some development, some potential for development, limited applicability to humans, limited suitability for large populations, questionable reproducibility, or questionable interpretability.

+ = Current information suggests adequate development, potential for further development applicable to humans, suitability for large populations, reproducibility, and interpretability.

++ = Current information suggests high development or good potential for substantial development, great applicability to humans, great suitability for large populations, reproducibility, or very good interpretability.

SOURCE: National Research Council, Subcommittee on Pulmonary Toxicology, *Biologic Markers in Pulmonary Toxicology* (Washington, DC: National Academy Press, 1989).

epidemiologic studies use FEV_1 as their measure of toxic effect in the large airways. Nitrogen washout tests have been used to measure small airways effects, but the sensitivity and specificity of that test has been called into question (29). Epidemiologists sometimes test for airway reactivity (28).

Bronchoalveolar lavage (BAL) could be performed in epidemiologic studies, either on living subjects or on autopsied lungs. BAL is invasive, however, and requires high-level skills to perform safely, adding to its expense and detracting from its utility in large-scale studies.

Assessments of data—Certain types of epidemiologic studies rely on routinely collected data rather than biological tests performed in the community. Death certificates provide mortality data that can be coupled with historical exposure data to draw some conclusions about the effects of inhaled pollutants on

a population. Morbidity data obtained from diverse sources—hospital admissions and discharge records (3,48), emergency room visits (33), hotline phone calls and follow-up interviews (5), reports of days lost from work or school—provide some indications about the effects of airborne toxicants as well. These sources may be affected by error. For instance, cause of death may be listed inaccurately; social and economic factors influence decisions to seek health care or miss work. Some epidemiologists believe that these errors tend to reduce (rather than increase) the possibility of finding a significant effect. Epidemiologists have relied on these types of information in studies that are widely accepted as indicative of a connection between exposure to inhaled substances and lung injury or disease.

Participants in epidemiologic studies of pulmonary toxicity often complete questionnaires to assess respiratory health (16). Quality control measures for standardized questionnaires have been assessed, and

---

Box 3-B—The UCLA Population Studies of Chronic Obstructive Respiratory Disease

In the early 1970s, researchers at the University of California at Los Angeles (UCLA) initiated a 10-part epidemiologic study of the respiratory effects of air pollution. By comparing the respiratory health of several communities exposed to different concentrations of common air pollutants, the researchers hoped to elucidate the connections between inhaled toxicants and chronic obstructive respiratory disease. The researchers chose Los Angeles as the study area because of the great variation in the types and concentrations of pollutants within a relatively small but highly populated geographical region. The existence of a uniform network of air quality monitoring stations throughout the area ensured the availability of exposure data, which also influenced the decision to perform the studies in the Los Angeles area.

Four Los Angeles area communities with similar demographics—Lancaster, Burbank, Long Beach, and Glendora—were chosen for study. Lancaster residents were exposed to relatively low levels of chemical air pollutants, while residents of Burbank, Long Beach, and Glendora were variously exposed to higher levels of chemical air pollutants including photochemical oxidants, sulfur dioxide, nitrogen dioxide, particulates, hydrocarbons, and sulfates.

For the initial part of the study, the investigators interviewed participants about respiratory symptoms, residence history, environmental and occupational exposures, and smoking history. Participants also performed lung function tests. The interviews and lung function tests were all performed at the same Mobile Lung Function Laboratory for which the reliability was determined and sensitivity and specificity were estimated. Though researchers noted that long-term studies were necessary, initial data led to the following hypotheses:

1. Adverse effects of long-term exposure to high concentrations of photochemical/oxidant pollutants may occur primarily in larger airways both among smokers and never smokers (comparisons of Lancaster and Burbank residents).

2. Long-term exposure to high concentrations of photochemical/oxidant pollutants and of sulfur dioxide, hydrocarbons, and particulate pollutants is associated with respiratory impairment, manifested by dysfunction of the large airways (comparisons of Lancaster, Burbank, and Long Beach residents).

3. Long-term exposure to high concentrations of photochemical oxidants, nitrogen dioxide, sulfates, and particulate pollutants may result in measurable impairment in lung function in smokers and never smokers (comparisons of Lancaster and Glendora residents).

Extensive follow-up enabled researchers to observe the populations from Lancaster, Burbank, Long Beach, and Glendora in long-term studies. Five years after the initial testing, participants still living in the study area (a substantial number) were reinterviewed and retested at the Mobile Lung Function Laboratory. These reexaminations lent support to the following hypotheses:

1. Chronic exposures to mixtures of photochemical oxidants, sulfates and particulates are associated with increased loss of lung function, which is especially evident in the small airways (comparison of Lancaster and Glendora residents.)

2. Chronic exposure to mixtures of sulfur dioxide, sulfates, oxides of nitrogen and/or hydrocarbons ultimately adversely affects the large airways as well as small airways (comparison of Lancaster and Long Beach residents).

3. Passive exposure to at least maternal smoking (but not to paternal smoking alone) affects the airways of younger boys (analysis of all four communities).

4. Smoking cessation leads to relatively early and sustained improvement in indexes of small airway function and other indices of respiratory health (analysis of all four communities).

The UCLA population studies of chronic obstructive respiratory disease add support to certain hypotheses regarding lung function and pollutant exposures. Nonetheless, the data reflect the types of problems that have characterized large epidemiologic studies. Exposure data are crude; experts fault the researchers controls for the effects of migration and self-selection. EPA concluded that the studies could not support standards setting for any of the pollutants involved. The studies do, however, point toward productive avenues for laboratory and clinical research that could clarify the effects of the pollutants found in the Los Angeles area on lung function.

SOURCE: Office of Technology Assessment, 1992, based on chapter 3 references 10,11,12,13,14,15,32,38,39,40,41,42.

---

though recall bias (sick or highly exposed individuals generally remember exposures or illnesses better than healthy or unexposed individuals) enters into play, questionnaires generally are considered useful. Daily diaries of short-term symptoms have become more prominent in recent years. They avoid the recall bias found in annual questionnaires and appear to be more sensitive (36).

Summary of Technologies Applicable to Epidemiologic Studies

In epidemiologic studies, exposure information is supplied with exposure assessment technologies and self-reported exposure data. Because "free-living" humans have knowing and unknowing encounters with multiple possible toxicants, exposure data in epidemiologic studies are necessarily imprecise. Many investigators believe that when confounding factors are properly accounted for, the ability to gather information on environmentally relevant exposures renders epidemiologic studies worthwhile even given the problems of collecting exposure data.

Biological tests applied in epidemiologic studies have the same advantages and disadvantages they present in laboratory and clinical studies, with the added requirement that they be easy to use in the field or on large populations. Reliance on public health records and population survey is a feature common to all epidemiology, including investigations of respiratory disease.

Summary of Health Effects Assessment Technologies

Each type of study (laboratory, clinical, or epidemiologic) has technological advantages and disadvantages, and individual studies within each type have strengths and weaknesses. Clear evidence of change in lung structure or function is unpersuasive if exposure data are problematic; evidence of health effects in animals under tightly conrolled exposure conditions may be unpersuasive if no human data are available. Despite the availability of many testing technologies, certainty about the pulmonary toxicity of many commercial substances has eluded investigators and regulators because of the lack of a full array of information sources. The database on the acute effects of short-term, high-dose exposures to toxicants is relatively large and growing, and forms the basis for existing regulations of pulmonary toxicants. Fewer data are available on the effects of chronic, "environmentally relevant" (i.e., low dose) exposures to suspected toxicants. On one hand, animal data on chronic exposures can be obtained using current testing technologies, but problems remain in extrapolating results from animals to humans. On the other hand, human data may be impractical or impossible to obtain given the ethical constraints of clinical testing and the length of time and large populations necessary to conduct meaningful epidemiologic studies.

LIMITS OF TECHNOLOGY

The previous sections establish that current technology can measure the biological effects of toxic substances on the lung, but that conclusion begs an important question: Are the measured effects adverse? Humans come equipped to survive in a hostile environment; most organ systems—the lung included—are resilient and operate with a reserve capacity that accommodates some level of change or damage (43). In the case of pulmonary toxicology, it appears science has learned to measure biological effects more quickly than it has learned to correlate those effects with persistent changes in performance or with disease processes. This disjuncture creates problems for regulators.

Most researchers recognize a hierarchy of biological effects of exposure to toxic substances, ranging from mortality (unarguably adverse) to measurable traces of toxicants in tissue (arguably adverse) (figure 3-3). Because some people or populations are more sensitive to toxic effects than others, and because some people or populations are more highly exposed to toxic substances than others, severe, unquestionably adverse effects are likely to occur in a smaller segment of the population than less severe, more questionably adverse effects. Effects may be reversible or irreversible, with a tendency among researchers to concern themselves more with irreversible effects. Concern for reversible effects increases, however, if chronic exposures prevent reversal. Evidence to support a clear demarcation between adverse and nonadverse effects remains elusive. If, as in the case of many suspected pulmonary toxicants, evidence does not exist to associate early changes with later, more extensive or irreversible changes, effects that are measurable may still be adjudged nonadverse.

The American Thoracic Society (ATS) has defined adverse respiratory health effects in humans as "medically significant physiologic or pathologic changes generally evidenced by one or more of the following: (1) interference with the normal activity of the affected person; (2) episodic respiratory illness; (3) incapacitating illness; (4) permanent respiratory injury; or (5) progressive respiratory dysfunction" (1). Most often, however, regulators must use a combination of limited

Figure 3-3—Spectrum of Biological Response to Pollutant Exposure

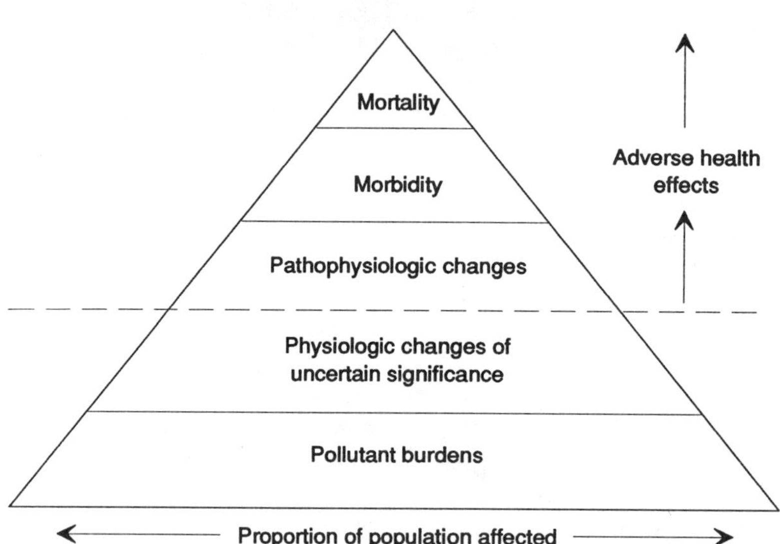

SOURCE: American Thoricic Society, "Guidelines as to What Constitutes an Adverse Respiratory Health Effect, with Special Reference to Epidemiologic Studies of Air Pollution,"*Am. Rev. Respir. Dis.* 131:666-668, 1985.

animal data and limited human data to reach conclusions about existing substances, and always must rely on animal data or extrapolations based on knowledge of chemical structures to predict the potential effects of new substances. Decisions about regulations most often are made in the absence of data that would enable a determination of adversity as precise as that found in the ATS definition.

Researchers and regulators agree that the integrated results of laboratory, clinical, and epidemiologic studies of short-term exposures can yield conclusive information about the acute effects of pulmonary toxicants. Current regulations generally are designed to prevent acute effects. Researchers and regulators generally are not satisfied that current technologies or current data provide them with a sufficient basis to regulate exposure to airborne toxicants because of the potential effects on the lung of chronic exposures. Much research is directed at developing improved methods for studying chronic exposures, but many questions remain. Chapter 4 provides more detail on regulations based on pulmonary toxicity and describes current Federal efforts to improve the basis for decision making with regard to chronic, low-dose exposure to inhaled toxics.

CHAPTER 3 REFERENCES

1. American Thoracic Society, "Guidelines as to What Constitutes an Adverse Respiratory Health Effect, With Special Reference to Epidemiologic Studies of Air Pollution," *American Review of Respiratory Disease* 131:666-668, 1985.

2. Barrow, C.S., "Generation and Characterization of Gases and Vapors," in *Concepts in Inhalation Toxicology,* R.O. McClellan and R.F. Henderson (eds.) (New York, NY: Hemisphere Publishing Corp., 1989), pp. 63-84.

3. Bates, D.V., and Sizto, R., "Air Pollution and Hospital Admissions in Southern Ontario: The Acid Summer Haze Effect," *Environmental Research* 43:317-331, 1987.

4. Becklake, M., McGill University, Montreal, Quebec, Canada, personal communication, September 1991.

5. Blanc, P.D., Galbo, M., Hiatt, P., et al., "Morbidity Following Acute Irritant Inhalation in a Population-Based Study," *Journal of the American Medical Association* 266(5):664-669, August 1991.

6. Cheng, Y.-S., and Moss, O.R., "Inhalation Exposure Systems," in *Concepts in Inhalation Toxicology,* R.O. McClellan and R.F. Henderson (eds.)

(New York, NY: Hemisphere Publishing Corp., 1989), pp. 19-62.

7. Costa, D.L., chief, Pulmonary Toxicology Branch, Health Effects Research Laboratory, EPA, Research Triangle Park, NC, personal communication, January 1992.

8. Dahl, A.R., Schlesinger, R.B., Heck, H.D'A., et al., "Comparative Dosimetry of Inhaled Materials: Differences Among Animal Species and Extrapolation to Man: Symposium Overview," *Fundamental and Applied Toxicology* 16:1-13, 1991.

9. Department of Health and Human Services, Task Force on Health Risk Assessment, *Determining Risks to Health: Federal Policy and Practice* (Dover, MA: Auburn House Publishing Company: MA, 1986).

10. Detels, R., Rokaw, S.N., Coulson, A.H., et al., " The UCLA Population Studies of Chronic Obstructive Respiratory Disease. I. Methodology and Comparison of Lung Function in Areas of High and Low Pollution," *American Journal of Epidemiology* 109(1):33-58, January 1979.

11. Detels, R., Sayre, J.W., Coulson, A.H., et al., "The UCLA Population Studies of Chronic Obstructive Respiratory Disease. IV. Respiratory Effect of Long-Term Exposure to Photochemical Oxidants, Nitrogen Dioxide, and Sulfates on Current and Never Smokers," *American Review of Respiratory Disease* 124(6):673-680, December 1981.

12. Detels, R., Sayre, J.W., Tashkin, D.P., et al., "The UCLA Population Studies of Chronic Obstructive Respiratory Disease. VI. Relationship of Physiologic Factors to Rate of Change in Forced Expiratory Volume in One Second and Forced Vital Capacity," *American Review of Respiratory Disease* 129(4):533-537, April 1984.

13. Detels, R., Tashkin, D.P., Sayre, J.W., et al., "The UCLA Population Studies of Chronic Obstructive Respiratory Disease. 9. Lung Function Changes Associated With Chronic Exposure to Photochemical Oxidants; A Cohort Study Among Never-Smokers," *Chest* 92(4):594-603, October 1987.

14. Detels, R., Tashkin, D.P., Sayre, J.W., et al., "The UCLA Population Studies of CORD: X. A Cohort Study of Changes in Respiratory Function Associated With Chronic Exposure to SO_x, NO_x, and Hydrocarbons," *American Journal of Public Health* 81(3):350-359, March 1991.

15. Detels, R., Tashkin, D.P., Simmons, M.S., et al., "The UCLA Population Studies of Chronic Obstructive Respiratory Disease. 5. Agreement and Disagreement of Tests in Identifying Abnormal Lung Function," *Chest* 82(5):630-638, November 1982.

16. Ferris, B.G., Jr., "Epidemiology Standardization Project," *American Review of Respiratory Disease* 118(Part 2):55-88, 1978.

17. Folinsbee, L.J., "Human Clinical Inhalation Exposures: Experimental Design, Methodology, and Physiological Responses," in *Toxicology of the Lung,* D.E. Gardner, et al. (eds.) (New York, NY: Raven Press, 1988), pp. 175-199.

18. Gehr, P., and Crapo, J.D., "Morphometric Analysis of the Gas Exchange Region of the Lung," in *Toxicology of the Lung*, D.E. Gardner, et al. (eds.) (New York, NY: Raven Press, 1988), pp. 1-42.

19. Haley, P.J., Finch, G.L., Hoover, M.D., et al., "The Acute Toxicity of Inhaled Beryllium Metal in Rats," *Fundamental and Applied Toxicology* 15:767-778, 1990.

20. Henderson, R.F., "Use of Bronchoalveolar Lavage to Detect Lung Damage," in *Toxicology of the Lung,* D.E. Gardner, et al. (eds.) (New York, NY: 1988), pp. 239-268.

21. Henderson, R.F., Benson, J.M., Hahn, F.F., et al., "New Approaches for the Evaluation of Pulmonary Toxicity: Bronchoalveolar Lavage Fluid Analysis," *Fundamental and Applied Toxicology* 5:451-458, 1985.

22. Lioy, P.J., "Assessing Total Human Exposure to Contaminants," *Environmental Science and Technology* 24(7):938-945, 1990.

23. Mauderly, J.L., "Comparisons of Respiratory Function Responses of Laboratory Animals and Humans," in *Inhalation Toxicology,* Mohr (ed.) (New York, NY: Springer-Verlag, 1988).

24. McClellan, R.O., "Health Effects of Diesel Exhaust: A Case Study in Risk Assessment," *American Industrial Hygienists Association Journal* 47(1):1-13, January 1986.

25. Mercer, R.R., and Crapo, J.D., "Structure of the Gas Exchange Region of the Lungs Determined by Three-Dimensional Reconstructions," in *Toxicology of the Lung,* D.E. Gardner, et al. (eds.) (New York, NY: Raven Press, 1988), pp. 117-146.

26. Moss, O.R., and Cheng, Y.-S., "Generation and Characterization of Test Atmospheres: Particles," in *Concepts in Inhalation Toxicology,* R.O.

McClellan and R.F. Henderson (eds.) (New York, NY: Hemisphere Publishing Corp., 1989), pp. 85-122.

27. National Research Council, *Risk Assessment in the Federal Government: Managing the Process* (Washington, DC: National Academy Press, 1983).

28. National Research Council, Committee on Epidemiology of Air Pollutants, *Epidemiology and Air Pollution* (Washington, DC: National Academy Press, 1985).

29. National Research Council, Subcommittee on Pulmonary Toxicology, *Biologic Markers in Pulmonary Toxicology* (Washington, DC: National Academy Press, 1989).

30. Overton, J.H., and Miller, F.J., "Absorption of Inhaled Reactive Gases," in *Toxicology of the Lung,* D.E. Gardner, et al. (eds.) (New York, NY: Raven Press, 1988), pp. 477-508.

31. Roggli, V.L., and Brody, A.R., "Imaging Techniques for Application to Lung Toxicology," in *Toxicology of the Lung,* D.E. Gardner, et al. (eds.) (New York, NY: Raven Press, 1988), pp. 117-146.

32. Rokaw, S.N., Detels, R., Coulson, A.H., et al., "The UCLA Population Studies of Chronic Obstructive Respiratory Disease. 3. Comparison of Pulmonary Function in Three Communities Exposed to Photochemical Oxidants, Multiple Primary Pollutants, or Minimal Pollutants," *Chest* 78(2):252-262, August 1980.

33. Samet, J.M., Bishop, Y., Speizer, F.E., et al., "The Relationship Between Air Pollution and Emergency Room Visits in an Industrial Community," *Journal of the Air Pollution Control Association* 31(3):236-240, March 1981.

34. Samet, J.M., and Utell, M.J., "The Environment and the Lung: Changing Perspectives," *Journal of the American Medical Association* 266(5):670-675, August 1991.

35. Schlesinger, R.B., "Biological Disposition of Airborne Particles: Basic Principles and Application to Vehicular Emissions," *Air Pollution, the Automobile, and Public Health* (Washington, DC: National Academy Press, 1988).

36. Schwartz, J., Environmental Protection Agency, Washington, DC, personal communication, January 1992.

37. Speizer, F., School of Public Health, Harvard University, Cambridge, MA, personal communication, December 1991.

38. Tashkin, D.P., Clark, V.A., Coulson, A.H., et al., "The UCLA Population Studies of Chronic Obstructive Respiratory Disease. VIII. Effects of Smoking Cessation on Lung Function: A Prospective Study of a Free-Living Population," *American Review of Respiratory Disease* 130(5):707-715, November 1984.

39. Tashkin, D.P., Clark, V.A., Simmons, M., et al., "The UCLA Population Studies of Chronic Obstructive Respiratory Disease. VII. Relationship Between Parental Smoking and Children's Lung Function," *American Review of Respiratory Disease* 129(6):891-897, June 1984.

40. Tashkin, D.P., Detels, R., Coulson, A.H., et al., "The UCLA Population Studies of Chronic Obstructive Respiratory Disease. II. Determination of Reliability and Estimation of Sensitivity and Specificity," *Environmental Research* 20(2):403-424, December 1979.

41. U.S. Environmental Protection Agency, "Air Quality Criteria for Ozone and Other Photochemical Oxidants," vol. 5, Environmental Criteria and Assessment Office, EPA/600/8-84/020bF, August 1986.

42. U.S. Environmental Protection Agency, Report of the Clean Air Science Advisory Committee (CASAC): "Review of the NAAQS for Ozone: Closure on the OAQPS Staff Paper (1988) and the Criteria Document Supplement (1988)," Office of the Administrator—Science Advisory Board, EPA-SAB-CASAC-89-019, Washington, DC, May 1989.

43. Utell, M.J., and Samet, J.M., "Environmentally Mediated Disorders of the Respiratory Tract," *Medical Clinics of North America* 74:291-306, March 1990.

44. Wagner, G., director, DRDS, National Institute for Occupational Safety and Health, Morgantown, WV, personal communication, January 1992.

45. Wallace, L.A., "The Total Exposure Assessment Methodology (TEAM) Study: Project Summary" (EPA/600/S6-87/002, September 1987).

46. Warheit, D.B., "Interspecies Comparisons of Lung Responses to Inhaled Particles and Gases," *Critical Reviews in Toxicology* 20(1):1-29, 1989.

47. Warheit, D.B., Carakostas, M.C., Hartsky, M.A., et al., "Development of a Short-Term Inhalation Bioassay to Assess Pulmonary Toxicity of Inhaled Particles: Comparisons of Pulmonary Responses to Carbonyl Iron and Silica," *Toxicology and Applied Pharmacology* 107:350-368, 1991.

48. Windau, J., Rosenman, K., Anderson, H., et al., "The Identification of Occupational Lung Disease From Hospital Discharge Data," *Journal of Occupational Medicine* 33(10):1060-1066, October 1991.

Chapter 4

Federal Attention to Pulmonary Toxicants

Federal Attention to Pulmonary Toxicants

INTRODUCTION

Congress has enacted a diverse body of laws to help control human exposure to toxicants. These laws require the Federal Government to regulate the public's exposure to toxic substances and to conduct and sponsor research that will improve identification and regulation of toxicants. This chapter describes regulatory and research programs of the Federal Government specifically related to the control and investigation of airborne pulmonary toxicants. The chapter provides examples of Federal activities but is not an exhaustive listing.

FEDERAL REGULATORY ACTIVITIES

Several Federal laws authorize administrative agencies to regulate substances to prevent adverse health effects, including respiratory effects. This section focuses on the laws and regulations used to control human exposures to pulmonary toxicants. The Environmental Protection Agency (EPA) and the Occupational Safety and Health Administration (OSHA), part of the Department of Labor (DOL), implement most of the statutes designed to limit human exposures to environmental and occupational pollutants. The Mine Safety and Health Administration (MSHA), also part of DOL, regulates pollution in the mining industry. The Consumer Product Safety Commission (CPSC) and the Food and Drug Administration (FDA) also have some authority over pulmonary toxicants.

Environmental Protection Agency

EPA administers a variety of laws that require protection of human health and the environment, including the Clean Air Act (CAA; 42 U.S.C. 7401 et seq.), the Resource Conservation and Recovery Act (RCRA; 42 U.S.C. 6901 et seq.), the Toxic Substances Control Act (TSCA; 15 U.S.C. 2601 et seq.), and the Federal Insecticide, Fungicide, and Rodenticide Act (FIFRA; 7 U.S.C. 136 et seq.). These statutes authorize EPA to control human exposure to substances that cause adverse human health effects, and the agency has, in fact, regulated some substances on the basis of pulmonary toxicity.

Clean Air Act

The CAA requires EPA to identify airborne substances that may "cause or contribute to air pollution which may reasonably be anticipated to endanger public health or welfare" and to set national ambient air quality standards (NAAQS) for those "criteria" pollutants. NAAQS, which apply only to outdoor concentrations of pollutants, have been set for sulfur oxides, particulate matter, carbon monoxide, ozone, nitrogen dioxide, and lead. EPA regulated sulfur oxides, particulate matter, ozone, and nitrogen dioxide because of their adverse effects on the pulmonary system (22,23). Table 4-1 presents the (health-based) primary ambient air quality standard for each criteria pollutant and lists adverse effects on the pulmonary system.

The CAA also requires EPA to control "hazardous air pollutants," defined by law as substances for which no ambient air quality standard can be set and that "may reasonably be anticipated to result in an increase in mortality or an increase in serious irreversible, or incapacitating reversible, illness." Between 1970 and 1984, seven substances were placed on the hazardous air pollutants list: asbestos, benzene, beryllium, inorganic arsenic, mercury, radionuclides, and vinyl chloride (3,23). Coke oven emissions were added to this list in 1984 (3). The 1990 amendments to the CAA substantially augmented the list of hazardous air pollutants—bringing it to 189—and required EPA to regulate them at the level possible under maximum achievable control technology (MACT) (23). Table 4-2 lists hazardous air pollutants known to be pulmonary toxicants.

Incentive Programs Under the CAA. Following adoption of the 1990 amendments to the CAA, EPA developed the Early Reduction Program (ERP), which provides incentives for companies to make immediate, major reductions (90 percent for gases and 95 percent

Table 4-1—National Primary Ambient Air Quality Standards

Pollutant	Primary standard	Effects on the lung
Sulfur oxides	80 micrograms/m^3 0.03 ppm annual arithmetic mean 0.14 ppm maximum 24-hour concentration not to be exceeded more than once a year	Can aggravate asthma, decrease lung function via inflammation; tendency develop allergies
Particulate matter	150 micrograms/m^3 24-hour average concentration 50 micrograms/m^3 annual arithmetic mean	Depending on specific particle, causes decreased lung function, bronchitis, and pneumonia; can aggravate asthma; some can cause fibrosis; increase deaths
Carbon monoxide	10 milligrams/m^3 9 ppm for an 8-hour average concentration not to exceed more than once a year 40 milligrams/m^3 35 ppm for a 1-hour average concentration not to be exceeded more than once a year	Can cause death or damage to lungcells by passing into the bloodstream inhibiting the ability of red blood cells to carry oxygen to cells of the body
Ozone	235 micrograms/m^3 0.12 ppm	Can irritate and inflame the lungs, cause shortness of breath, increased susceptibility to respiratory infections, accelerated aging of the lungs, and emphysema; fatal at high concentrations (effects have been shown below the current standard
Nitrogen dioxide	100 micrograms/m^3 0.053 ppm annual arithmetic mean concentration	Can cause acute respiratory disease at high concentrations, increased susceptibility to viral infections; can aggravate asthma; can cause inflammation
Lead	1.5 micrograms/m^3 maximum arithmetic mean averaged over a calendar quarter	Lung acts as site of entry for lead which in turn can damage the nervous system, kidneys, and reproductive system

SOURCES: 40 CFR 50, July 1, 1991; U.S. Congress, *United States Code Congressional and Administrative News, 95th Congress, 1st Sess. 1977* (St. Paul, MN: West Publishing Co., 1977), pp. 1187-88; U.S. Congress, *United States Code Congressional and Administrative News, 101st Congress, 2d Sess., 1990* (St. Paul, MN: West Publishing Co., 1990), pp. 3392-94.

for particulates) in their emissions of hazardous air pollutants. Companies that participate in the ERP will be allowed a 6-year compliance extension after emissions standards (anticipated to require reductions in excess of 90 to 95 percent) are developed. EPA monitors company compliance with the ERP and focuses on specific sources, even sources within a plant's boundaries. Participating companies who fail to make the voluntary reductions will not receive the compliance extension (24).

The ERP covers all 189 hazardous air pollutants listed in the CAA, but it identifies 35 substances deemed "highly toxic pollutants" as its most important targets. Each of these substances is weighted according to its toxicity, and volume and total toxicity must both be reduced in order to fulfill the requirements of the ERP (24). Table 4-3 lists substances covered by the ERP that are known to be pulmonary toxicants.

EPA also designed the 33/50 Program to encourage companies to make voluntary reductions in pollutant emissions before MACT standards are in place. The 33/50 Program asks companies to voluntarily reduce aggregate releases and off site transfers of 17 high priority toxic substances by a total of 33 percent by 1992 and a total of 50 percent by 1995. This program does not focus on reducing emissions at or within particular plants but concentrates on national goals (25).

Each substance covered by the 33/50 Program:

- appears on the CAA's list of hazardous air pollutants;
- is included in the Toxic Release Inventory (TRI);
- is a multimedia pollutant on the agenda of every department of EPA;
- is produced in large quantities and has a high release to production ratio;
- has been shown to be amenable to pollution control; and
- is known to be toxic to both human health and the environment (8).

Table 4-3 lists the chemicals targeted by the 33/50 Program that are known to be pulmonary toxicants. Participants in the 33/50 Program set their own goals for emissions reductions, and EPA has no enforcement mechanism. Compliance is measured through TRI reporting and is not as closely monitored as in the ERP (24).

Resource Conservation and Recovery Act

RCRA attempts to safeguard public health and the environment by controlling waste disposal. It requires EPA to identify and list hazardous wastes, defined as solid wastes, which due to potency, volume, or physical, chemical, or infectious qualities may:

- cause or considerably add to deaths or serious irreversible or incapacitating reversible illness, or
- create significant present or potential dangers to human and environmental health if improperly handled.

Several chemicals regulated under RCRA have adverse effects on the pulmonary system; see table 4-4.

Toxic Substances Control Act

TSCA calls on EPA to regulate chemicals in pre-marketing and post-marketing phases to avoid unreasonable risk of injury to public health and the environment. TSCA requires the manufacturer to provide EPA with a pre-manufacturing notice (PMN), including test results on the chemical, at least 90 days before manufacturing begins. If EPA does not request further data within the 90-day period, the manufacturer is free to begin production (2). If EPA finds that the chemical may pose an unreasonable risk to human health or the environment, or that insufficient data exist to make a determination about risk, or that the chemical will be produced in substantial quantities, EPA may require additional testing. This testing is conducted by the chemical manufacturer or processor.

Many of the regulations issued under TSCA (40 CFR 790 et seq.) provide guidelines for testing chemicals. Guidelines exist for testing acute, sub-chronic, and chronic inhalation toxicity. Acute inhalation toxicity testing provides information on health hazards likely to result from short-term exposure to a substance. Acute inhalation tests involve a single, 4- to 24-hour exposure to a particular substance followed by a 14-day observation period. The sub-chronic inhalation tests assess the effects of toxicants from repeated daily exposures to a substance for approximately 10 percent of the animal's lifespan. These tests involve repeated daily exposures for at least 90 days. Chronic toxicity inhalation testing is designed to determine the health effects that are cumulative or have a long latency period. These tests involve repeated daily exposures to a substance for at least 12 months.

If tests show that a chemical poses an unreasonable risk to human health or the environment, EPA can limit or prohibit its use, manufacture, and distribution. EPA has taken action under TSCA due to the possibility that certain chemicals pose pulmonary health threats. For example, EPA has required manufacturers to report health and safety study data on 26 diisocyanates because of concern that acute and chronic exposures could cause respiratory tract effects and nose irritation (5). EPA has also required significant new use evaluations for substituted oxirane, substituted al-

Table 4-2—Hazardous Air Pollutants Regulated Under the CAA Due to Non-Cancer Health Effects on the Pulmonary System

Chemical	Pulmonary health effect
Acetaldehyde	Respiratory tract irritation
Acrolein	Respiratory tract irritation
Acrylic acid	Lung injury, and possibly death
Allyl chloride	Pulmonary irritation and histologic lesions of the lung
Asbestos	Asbestosis
Benzene	Pulmonary edema and hemorrhage; tightness in chest, breathlessness; unconsciousness may occur and death may follow due to respiratory paralysis in cases of extreme exposure
Benzyl chloride	Lung damage and pulmonary edema
Beryllium compounds	Non-malignant respiratory disease and berylliosis
Caprolactam	Upper respiratory tract irritation and congestion
Catechol	Acute respiratory toxicity and upper respiratory tract irritation
Chlorine	Necrosis of tracheal and bronchial epithelium, bronchitis, bronchopneumonia and fatal pulmonary edema
2-Chloroacetophenone	Difficulty in breathing
Chloroprene	Lung irritation
Chromium	Pulmonary disease (unspecified)
Cresol (o-, m-, & p-)	Obliterative bronchiolitis, ademonatosis, and hypersentivity reactions, chronic interstitial pneumonitis and occasional fatalities
Diazomethane	Chest pain, respiratory irritation, damages to mucous membranes
Dichloroethyl ether	Respiratory system irritation and pulmonary damage
1,3-Dichloropropene	Respiratory irritation
Dimethyl sulfate	Lung edema
2,4-Dinitrophenol	Respiratory collapse
1,4-Dioxane (1,4-Diethleneoxide)	Lung edema; can cause death
1,2-Epoxybutane	Lung irritation, edema, and pneumonitis
Epichlorohydrin	Lung edema, dyspnea, bronchitis, and throat irritation
Ethyl acrylate	Respiratory irritation, pneumonia and pulmonary edema
Ethyl benzene	Lung congestion
Ethylene glycol	Throat and respiratory irritation
Ethylene imine (Aziridine)	Lung edema and secondary bronchial pneumonia
Ethylene oxide	Respiratory irritation and lung injury (unspecified)
Formaldehyde	Difficulty breathing, severe respiratory tract injury leading to pulmonary edema, pneumonitis, and bronchial irritation which may lead to death
Hexachlorobutadiene	Pulmonary irritation
Hexachlorocyclopentadiene	Pulmonary irritation, bronchitis, and bronchiolitis
Hexamethylene-1,6-diisocyanate	Pulmonary edema, chronic bronchitis, chronic asthma; pulmonary edema; may be fatal

Table 4-2—Hazardous Air Pollutants Regulated Under the CAA Due to Non-Cancer Health Effects on the Pulmonary System (Cont'd)

Chemical	Pulmonary health effect
Hydrochloric acid	Pulmonary edema
Hydrogen fluoride	Respiratory tract irritation and lung damage
Hydrogen sulfide	Pulmonary edema
Maleic anhydride	Chronic bronchitis
Methyl bromide	Bronchopneumonia
Methyl ethyl ketone	Upper respiratory tract irritation
Methyl iodide (Iodomethane)	Lung irritation
Methyl isocyanate	Pulmonary edema and lung injury
Methyl methacrylate	Fatal pulmonary edema
Methylene diphenyl diisocyanate (MDI)	Restricted pulmonary function
Napthalene	Lung damage
2-Nitropropane	Pulmonary edema
p-Phenylenediamine	Allergic asthma and inflammation of larynx and pharynx
Phosgene	Extreme lung damage; severe pulmonary edema after a latent period of exposure; bleeding and painful breathing; death
Phosphine	Pulmonary edema and acute dyspnea
Phthalic anhydride	Respiratory irritation and pulmonary sensitization
Propionaldehyde	Fatal pulmonary edema
Propoxur (Baygon)	Severe bronchoconstriction and paralysis of respiratory muscles
Propylene oxide	Pulmonary irritation
1,2-Propylenimine (2-Methyl aziridine)	Diphtheria-like mutations of trachea and bronchi; bronchitis, lung edema, secondary bronchial pneumonia
Styrene	Abnormal pulmonary function, upper respiratory tract irritation, wheezing, chest tightness, and shortness of breath
Tetrachloroethylene (Perchloroethylene)	Acute pulmonary edema
2,4-Toluene diisocyanate	Pulmonary sensitization and long-term decline in lung function
Toxaphene (Chlorinated camphene)	Lung inflammation
1,2,4-Trichlorobenzene	Lung and upper respiratory tract irritation
Trichloroethylene	Lung adenomas
Triethylamine	Vapors cause severe coughing, difficulty breathing, and chest pain; pulmonary edema
2,2,4-Trimethylpentane	Pulmonary lesions
Vinyl acetate	Upper respiratory tract irritation

SOURCES: 42 U.S.C. 7412; Tim Simpson, U.S. Environmental Protection Agency, Research Triangle Park, NC, personal communication, August 1991; 54 *Federal Register* 2329-2984 (Jan. 19, 1989).

Table 4-3—Pulmonary Toxicants Controlled Under EPA's Early Reduction and 33/50 Programs

Early Reduction Program	Effect
Asbestos	Asbestosis
Acrolein	Respiratory irritation
Acrylic acid	Lung injury and possible death
Benzene	Pulmonary edema and hemmorhage; tightness of chest, breathlessness; unconsciousness may occur and death may follow due to paralysis in cases of extreme exposure
Beryllium compounds	Non-malignant respiratory disease and berylliosis
Chloroprene	Lung irritation
Chromium compounds	Pulmonary disease and other toxic effects
Dichloroethyl ether	Respiratory system irritation and damage
Methyl isocyanate	Pulmonary edema
Methylene diphenyl diisocyanate (MDI)	Restricted pulmonary function
Phosgene	Extreme lung damage; severe pulmonary edema after a latent period of exposure; bleeding and painful breathing; death
2,4 Toluene diisocyanate	Pulmonary sensitization and long-term decline in lung function

33/50 Program	Effect
Benzene	Pulmonary edema and hemmorhage; tightness of chest, breathlessness and unconsciousness may occur and death may follow due to respiratory paralysis in cases of extreme exposure
Chromium & chromium compounds	Pulmonary disease and other toxic effects
Methyl ethyl ketone	Upper respiratory tract irritation
Nickel & nickel compounds	Pulmonary irritation, pulmonary damage, hyperplasia, and interstitial fibrotic lesions
Tetrachloroethylene	Acute pulmonary edema
Trichloroethylene	Lung adenomas

SOURCES: U.S. Environmental Protection Agency, Office of Air and Radiation, "Early Reduction Program," unpublished memo, Washington, DC, July 1991; U.S. Environmental Protection Agency, "EPA's 33/50 Program: A Progress Report," unpublished memo, Washington, DC, July 1991; Tim Simpson, U.S. Environmental Protection Agency, Research Triangle Park, NC, personal communication, August 1991; 54 *Federal Register* 2329-2984 (Jan. 19, 1989).

kyl halides, and perhalo alkoxy ether due to the threat of pulmonary edema. EPA imposed the same requirement on silane because data showed that it causes irreversible lung toxicity (6).

Federal Insecticide, Fungicide, and Rodenticide Act

FIFRA was enacted to help avoid unreasonable adverse effects on the environment, including humans, due to exposure to pesticides. It requires those who sell or distribute pesticides to register the product with EPA. A product may be classified and registered for general or restricted use, or both. If a pesticide is classified for restricted use because it poses an inhalation toxicity hazard to the applicator or other persons, then the product may only be applied by or used under the direct supervision of a certified applicator. Substances that pose inhalation hazards are substances that are dangerous to some organ and that enter the body through the lung. Not all inhalable toxicants af-

Table 4-4—Regulated Levels of Pulmonary Toxicants Under RCRA

Contaminant	Pulmonary effect	Regulatory level (mg/L)
Arsenic	Respiratory irritation and inflammation	5.0
Benzene	Pulmonary edema and hemmorhage; tightness of chest, breathlessness and unconsciousness may occur and death may follow due to respiratory paralysis in cases of extreme exposure	0.5
Chromium	Pulmonary disease and other toxic effects	5.0
Cresol (o-, m- & p-)	Obliterative broncholitis, adenomatosis, and hypersensitivity reactions; chronic interstitial pneumonitis and occasional fatalities	200.0
Methyl ethyl ketone	Upper respiratory tract irritation	200.0
Tetrachloroethylene	Acute pulmonary edema	0.7
Toxaphene	Lung inflammation	0.5

SOURCES: 40 CFR 261.24, July 1, 1991; Tim Simpson, U.S. Environmental Protection Agency, Research Triangle Park, NC, personal communication, August 1991; 54 *Federal Register* 2329-2984 (Jan. 19, 1989).

Table 4-5—Pulmonary Toxicants Regulated Under FIFRA

Active ingredient in pesticide	Criteria influencing restriction
Acrolein	Respiratory tract irritant
Allyl alcohol	Upper respiratory tract irritant
Hydrocyanic acid	Upper respiratory tract irritant
Methyl bromide	Lung irritant; causes pulmonary edema
Methyl parathion	Excessive exposure may cause bronchoconstriction
Paraquat (dichloride) and paraquat bis(methyl sulfate)	Pulmonary irritant; can cause pulmonary edema, intra-alveolar hemmorhage, and death

SOURCES: 40 CFR 152.175, July 1, 1991; 54 *Federal Register* 2329-2984 (Jan. 19, 1989).

fect the lung; table 4-5 lists active pesticide ingredients regulated under FIFRA that are pulmonary toxicants.

Department of Labor

Two entities within DOL regulate human exposure to airborne toxicants. OSHA administers the Occupational Safety and Health Act (OSH Act; 29 U.S.C. 651 et seq.). MSHA administers the Federal Mine Safety and Health Act (FMSHA; 30 U.S.C. 801), which operates similarly to the OSH Act but is restricted to the mining industry.

Occupational Safety and Health Administration

OSHA's task is to develop regulations for the use of toxic substances in the workplace. OSHA can require specific handling procedures, training for workers, recordkeeping, and testing of hazardous materials. It can also establish or modify permissible exposure limits (PELs) for toxic substances. Many substances are regulated by OSHA because of their detrimental effects on the pulmonary system. Table 4-6 lists air contaminants regulated by OSHA because of pulmonary toxicity.

Table 4-6—Air Contaminants Regulated by OSHA Because of Pulmonary Effects

Substance	Effects
Acetyladehyde	Respiratory tract irritation
Acetic acid	Bronchial constriction, respiratory tract irritation, bronchitis, and pharyngitis
Acetic anhydride	Nose and throat irritation; bronchial and lung irritation
Acetone	Pharyngial and lung irritation; inflammation of respiratory tract; irritation and infections of respiratory tract
Acetylsalicyclic acid	Respiratory tract irritation
Acrolein	Respiratory irritation
Acrylic acid	Lung injury and possible death
Allyl alcohol	Upper respiratory tract irritation
Allyl chloride	Histologic lesions of the lung and pulmonary irritation
Allyl glycidyl ether	Respiratory irritation
Allyl propyl disulfide	Upper respiratory tract irritation
Aluminum	Pulmonary fibrosis and respiratory irritation
Ammonia	Upper respiratory tract irritation
Ammonium chloride fume	Respiratory tract irritation
Arsenic	Respiratory irritation and inflammation
Asbestos	Causes asbestosis
Barium sulfate	Upper respiratory tract irritation and pneumoconiosis
Benzene	Pulmonary edema and hemorrhage; tightness of chest, breathlessness; unconsciousness may occur and death may follow due to respiratory paralysis in cases of extreme exposure
Benzyl chloride	Shown to cause lung damage and pulmonary edema in animals
Beryllium & beryllium compounds	Non-malignant respiratory disease and berylliosis
Bismuth telluride	Granulomatous lesions in lungs
Borates	Upper respiratory tract irritation
Boron oxide	Upper respiratory tract irritation
Boron tribromide	Pneumonia and pneumonitis
Bromine	Respiratory tract irritation and lung edema
2-Butoxyethanol	Toxic lung changes
n-Butyl acetate	Respiratory irritation
n-Butyl lactate	Upper respiratory tract irritation
o-sec-Butylphenol	Respiratory tract irritation
Calcium hydroxide	Severe caustic irritation to upper respiratory tract
Calcium oxide	Inflammation of respiratory tract and pneumonia
Camphor	Inflammation of upper respiratory tract; dyspnea
Caprolactam	Congestion and irritation of upper respiratory tract
Captofol (Difolatan)	Respiratory sensitization
Carbonyl fluoride	Respiratory tract irritation
Catechol	Acute respiratory toxicity and upper respiratory tract irritation
Cesium hydroxide	Respiratory tract irritation
Chlorine	Necrosis of tracheal and bronchial epithelium, bronchitis, bronchopneumonia and fatal pulmonary edema
Chlorine dioxide	Respiratory irritation and bronchitis
a-Chloroacetophenone	Difficulty in breathing
Chloroacetyl chloride	Respiratory irritation, cough, dyspnea, and pulmonary edema

Table 4-6—Air Contaminants Regulated by OSHA Because of Pulmonary Effects (Cont'd)

Substance	Effects
o-Chlorobenzylidene malononitrile	Upper respiratory tract irritation and dyspnea
Chromium metal	Pulmonary disease (unspecified)
Coal dust (greater and less than 5 percent quartz)	Pneumoconiosis and fibrosis after long-term exposure
Cobalt (metal, dust, and fume)	Obliterative bronchiolitis adenomatosis, asthma, and chronic interstitial pneumonia
Cobalt carbonyl	Coughing and dyspnea
Cobalt hydrocarbonyl	Lung damage (unspecified)
Cotton dust	Byssinosis
Cresol (all isomers)	Obliterative bronchiolitis; adenomatosis; hypersensitivity reactions; chronic interstitial pneumonitis and occasional fatalities
Cyanogen chloride	Pulmonary edema and upper respiratory tract irritation
Cyclohexanone	Respiratory tract irritation
Cyhexatin	Respiratory irritation
1,2-dibromo-3-chloropropane	Upper respiratory tract irritation
Dibutyl phosphate	Respiratory tract irritation
Dichloroacetylene	Pulmonary edema
Dicholorethyl ether	Lung injury (unspecified)
1,3-dichloropropene	Respiratory irritation
2,2-dichloropropionic acid	Respiratory irritation
Dicyclopentadiene	Respiratory irritation and lung hemorrhage
Diethylamine	Tracheitis, bronchitis, pneumonitis, and pulmonary edema
Diethylene triamine	Respiratory tract sensitization
Diglycidyl ether	Respiratory irritation
Diisobutyl ketone	Upper respiratory tract irritation
Dimethyl sulfate	Lung edema
Dioxane	Pulmonary edema; can cause death through repeated exposures at low concentrations
Divinyl benzene	Respiratory irritation
Emery	Respiratory tract irritation and pneumonconisis
Epichlorohydrin	Lung edema, respiratory tract irritation, dyspnea, and bronchitis
Ethanoamine	Lung damage (unspecified)
Ethyl acrylate	Respiratory irritation, pneumonia and pulmonary edema
Ethyl benzene	Lung congestion
Ethyl bromide	Respiratory tract irritation; lung irritation and congestion
Ethyl silicate	Lung damage (unspecified)
Ethylene chlorohydrin	Respiratory tract and lung irritation
Ethylene glycol	Respiratory tract irritation
Ethylene imine	Lung edema and secondary bronchial pneumonia
Ethylene oxide	Respiratory irritation and lung injury (unspecified)
Ferbam	Upper respiratory tract irritation
Ferrovanadium dust	Chronic bronchitis and chronic lung inflammation
Formaldehyde	Difficulty breathing, severe respiratory tract injury leading to pulmonary edema, pneumonitis, and bronchial irritation which may lead to death depending on concentration of exposure; chronic exposure may lead to development of bronchitis and asthma

Table 4-6—Air Contaminants Regulated by OSHA Because of Pulmonary Effects (Cont'd)

Substance	Effects
Furfural	Respiratory tract irritation
Furfuryl alcohol	Asthma
Gluteraldehyde	Upper respiratory tract irritation
Glycidol	Respiratory tract and lung irritation, pneumonitis and emphysema
Grain dust (oat, wheat, barley)	Chronic bronchitis, asthma, dyspnea, wheezing, and reduced pulmonary function
Graphite	Pneumoconosis and anthracosilicosis
Hexachlorobutadiene	Pulmonary irritation
Hexachlorocyclopentadiene	Pulmonary irritation, bronchitis, and bronchiolitis
Hexalene glycol	Respiratory irritation
Hydrogen bromide	Upper respiratory tract irritation
Hydrogen cyanide	Upper respiratory tract irritation and dyspnea
Hydrogen fluoride	Respiratory tract irritation
Hydrogen sulfide	Pulmonary edema; fatal at high concentrations
Hydrogenated terphenyls	Lung damage (unspecified)
Indene	Chemical pneumonitis, pulmonary edema and lung hemorrhage
Indium & Indium compounds	Widespread alveolar edema
Iron oxide	Siderosis
Iron pentacarbonyl	Pulmonary injury and dyspnea
Isoamyl alcohol	Upper respiratory tract irritation
Isophorone diisocyanate	Respiratory tract irritation, decreased pulmonary function, and sensitization
n-Isopropylamine	Respiratory tract irritation
Isopropy glycidyl ether	Upper respiratory tract irritation
Kaolin	Respiratory effects (unspecified)
Ketene	Respiratory tract irritation and pulmonary edema
Limestone	Upper respiratory tract irritation
Magnesium oxide fume	Chronic respiratory disease (unspecified)
Maleic anhydride	Chronic bronchitis
Manganese cyclopentadienyl tricarbonyl	Pulmonary edema
Manganese fume	Pneumonia and lung damage (unspecified)
Manganese tetroxide	Pneumonitis and other respiratory effects
Methyl acetate	Pulmonary irritation
Methyl bromide	Bronchopneumonia, lung irritation, and pulmonary edema
Methyl demeton	Lung congestion
Methyl ethyl ketone	Upper respiratory tract irritation
Methyl ethyl ketone peroxide	Upper respiratory tract irritation and lung damage (unspecified)
Methyl formate	Pulmonary edema, lung inflammation, and dyspnea
Methyl iodide	Lung irritation
Methyl isocyanate	Pulmonary edema and lung irritation
Methyl mercaptan	Pulmonary edema
Methyl methacrylate	Fatal pulmonary edema
Methyl parathion	Bronchioconstriction
Methylcyclohexanol	Respiratory irritation
Methylene bis(4-cyclohexylisocyanate)	Pulmonary irritation

Table 4-6—Air Contaminants Regulated by OSHA Because of Pulmonary Effects (Cont'd)

Substance	Effects
Mica	Symptoms resembling those of silicosis and pneumoconiosis
Morpholine	Thickened alveoli, emphysema, and respiratory irritation
Nickel (soluble compounds)	Pulmonary irritation, interstitial fibrotic lesions, hyperplasia
Nitric acid	Chronic bronchitis and pneumonitis
Nitrogen dioxide	Chronic bronchitis, emphysema, and decreased lung capacity
2-Nitropropane	Pulmonary edema from severe exposure
Oil mist (mineral)	Respiratory tract irritation
Osmium tetroxide	Respiratory irritation
Oxalic acid	Respiratory tract irritation
Oxygen difluoride	Pulmonary edema and hemorrhage
Ozone	Significant reduction in pulmonary vital capacity and pulmonary congestion
Paraquat	Pulmonary irritation, pulmonary edema, and intra-alveolar hemorrhage
Particulates (not otherwise regulated)	Upper respiratory tract irritation
Perchloryl fluoride	Alveolar hemorrhage, emphysema, and alveolar edema
Phenol	Guinea pigs died after inhalation exposure; no human inhalation data
Phenyl glycidyl ether	Respiratory tract irritation
p-Phenylenediamine	Allergic asthma and inflammation of the larynx and pharynx from industrial exposure
Phenylhydrazine	Lung adenomas
Phenyl mercaptan	Lung toxicity
Phosgene	Extreme lung damage; severe pulmonary edema after latent period of exposure; bleeding and painful breathing; causes death
Phosphine	Pulmonary edema and acute dyspnea; at concentrations of 400 to 600 pm death may occur 30 minutes to 1 hour after exposure
Phosphoric acid	Respiratory irritation
Phosphorous oxychloride	Respiratory tract irritation and pulmonary edema
Phosphorous pentasulfide	Respiratory irritation
Phosphorous trichloride	Bronchitis and pneumonia
Phthalic anhydride	Respiratory irritation and pulmonary sensitization
Picric acid	Edema, papules, vesicles, and desquamations of the nose
Piperazine dihydrochloride	Pulmonary sensitization
Portland cement	Respiratory irritation
Potassium hydroxide	Respiratory irritation
Propionic acid	Respiratory tract irritation
n-Propyl acetate	Respiratory irritation
Propylene oxide	Respiratory irritation
Rhodium compounds	Respiratory sensitization
Rosin core solder pyrolysis products	Upper respiratory tract irritation
Rouge	Upper respiratory tract irritation
Silica	Silicosis
Silicon	Pulmonary lesions
Silicon carbide	Aggravates pulmonary tuberculosis
Silicon tetrahydride	Upper respiratory tract irritation
Soapstone	Pneumoconiosis

Table 4-6—Air Contaminants Regulated by OSHA Because of Pulmonary Effects (Cont'd)

Substance	Effects
Sodium azide	Bronchitis
Sodium bisulfite	Respiratory irritation
Sodium hydroxide	Upper respiratory tract irritation and pneumonitis
Stoddard solvent	Lung congestion and emphysema
Styrene	Upper respiratory tract irritation and abnormal pulmonary function
Subtilisins	Bronchoconstrictions and respiratory tract irritation
Sulfur dioxide	Accelerated loss of pulmonary function, bronchoconstriction, and dyspnea
Sulfur monochloride	Lung irritation
Sulfur pentafluoride	Lung congestion, lesions, and pulmonary edema
Sulfur tetrafluoride	Emphysema, pulmonary edema, and difficulty breathing
Sulfuryl fluoride	Pulmonary edema
Talc	Pneumoconiosis, pleural thickening and calcification, reduced pulmonary function, and fibrotic changes in lung tissue
Tantalum	Lung lesions, bronchitis, hyperemia, and interstitial pneumonitis
Terphenyls	Respiratory tract irritation
Tetrachloroethylene	Long-term decline in lung function and pulmonary edema
Tetrasodium pyrophosphate	Respiratory tract irritation
Tin oxide	Stannosis and reduced pulmonary capacity
Toluene-2,4-diisocyanate	Pulmonary sensitization and long term decline in lung function
Toxaphene	Lung inflammation
Tributyl phosphate	Lung toxicity
1,2,4-Trichlorobenzene	Upper respiratory tract irritation
1,2,3-Trichloropropane	Upper respiratory tract irritation
Triethylamine	Pulmonary irritation
Trimellitic anhydride	Intra-alveolar hemorrhage
Trimethyl phosphite	Lung irritation
Trimethylamine	Upper respiratory tract irritation
Trimethylbenzene	Asthmatic bronchitis
Tungsten & tungsten compounds (insoluble)	Proliferation of intra-alveolar septa, pulmonary fibrosis, and dyspnea
Vanadium dust	Bronchial irritation and tracheobronchitis
Vanadium fume	Bronchitis, emphysema, tracheitis, pulmonary edema, and bronchial pneumonia
Vinyl acetate	Upper respiratory tract irritation
VM&P Naphtha	Upper respiratory tract irritation
Welding fumes	Damage to small airways causing interstial pneumonia; respiratory irritation
Wood dust	Allergic respiratory effects, decrease in pulmonary function
Zinc chloride fume	Damage to respiratory tract, severe pneumonitis, and advanced pulmonary fibrosis
Zinc oxide fume	Shortness of breath and pneumonia
Zinc oxide dust	Respiratory effects (unspecified)
Zinc stearate	Pulmonary fibrosis
Zirconium compounds	Granulomas in the lung

SOURCES: 29 CFR 1910.1000, July 1, 1991; 29 CFR 1910.1001, July 1, 1991; 29 CFR 1910.1018, July 1, 1991; 29 CFR 1910.1028, July 1, 1991; 29 CFR 1910.1044, July 1, 1991; 29 CFR 1910.1043, July 1, 1991; 29 CFR 1910.1044, July 1, 1991; 29 CFR 1910.1047, July 1, 1991; 29 CFR 1910.1048, July 1, 1991; 53 *Federal Register* 21062 (June 7, 1988); 54 *Federal Register* 2329-2984 (Jan. 19, 1989).

Mine Safety and Health Administration

MSHA develops regulations to protect the health and safety of miners. It administers FMSHA, which is clearly concerned about pulmonary toxicants. FMSHA uses the framework for health guidelines presented in the Federal Coal Mine Health and Safety Act of 1969, which was primarily concerned with black lung disease, a form of pneumoconiosis common to coal miners (21,22). The statute and regulations require air sampling, medical examinations for miners, and dust control measures. A stated purpose of the health standards was to ensure that mines are "sufficiently free of respirable dust concentrations . . . to permit each miner the opportunity to work underground during the period of his entire adult working life without incurring any disability from pneumoconiosis or any other occupation-related disease during or at the end of such period."

Other Federal Regulatory Activities

EPA and DOL exercise the main regulatory authority over airborne pulmonary toxicants. Other agencies also administer laws that can be used to control these substances, however. CPSC enforces the Consumer Product Safety Act (CPSA; 15 U.S.C. 2051 et seq.) and the Federal Hazardous Substances Act (FHSA; 15 U.S.C. 1261 et seq.). The FDA regulates chemicals found in foods, drugs and cosmetics under the Federal Food, Drug, and Cosmetic Act (FDCA; 21 U.S.C. 301 et seq.).

Consumer Product Safety Commission

The CPSC conducts research on injuries and diseases caused by consumer products and disperses information. The commission is also charged with the duty of generating consumer product safety standards and monitoring compliance.

Consumer Product Safety Act—CSPA is intended to protect the American public from undue risk of injury from consumer products and to help consumers judge the comparative safety of articles available in the marketplace. CPSA gives CPSC the authority to ban or recall hazardous products. Few regulations issued under CPSA (16 CFR 1000 et seq.) deal specifically with health hazards to the pulmonary system posed by unsafe consumer products. However, several products containing asbestos are mentioned specifically as banned materials. Consumer patching compounds containing respirable free-form asbestos are prohibited on the American market. Also, artificial emberizing materials (e.g., artificial fireplace logs) containing respirable free-form asbestos are forbidden. The regulations for these products specify the reason for the ban as the unreasonable risk of lung cancer, noncancerous lung diseases and injury due to inhaling asbestos fibers.

Federal Hazardous Substances Act. FHSA is intended to protect the public from health problems by requiring that hazardous substances be labeled to warn individuals of associated health risks. Regulations issued under FHSA control a number of pulmonary toxicants, including formaldehyde, which is a strong sensitizer (a substance that causes normal living tissue, through an allergic or photodynamic process, to become severely hypersensitive on re-exposure to the substance).

The regulations also control "hazardous substances," which are defined as materials that have the potential to cause substantial personal injury or substantial illness as a result of any customary or reasonably foreseeable use or handling. Benzene, products containing 5 percent or more by weight of benzene, and products containing 10 percent or more by weight of toluene, xylene, turpentine, or petroleum distillates (e.g., kerosene, naphtha, and gasoline) are listed as hazardous substances. Such products must be clearly labeled with several words and symbols including "danger" and "harmful or fatal if swallowed" since these materials may be aspirated into the lungs causing chemical pneumonitis, pneumonia, and pulmonary edema.

Food and Drug Administration

FDA regulates chemicals found in foods, drugs, and cosmetics, primarily through FDCA. Some of FDA's actions under this statute have been taken to protect pulmonary health. For example, sulfites are subject to a number of FDA regulatory requirements because they have been found to cause severe, and potentially lethal, asthma attacks in sensitive individuals. Sulfites are no longer considered safe for use in meats, fruits and vegetables to be served or sold raw or presented to consumers as fresh (21 CFR 182). The presence of sulfites in food must be declared when these chemicals are present at levels above 10 parts per million. However, FDA has not regulated airborne substances because of pulmonary toxicity.

FEDERAL RESEARCH ACTIVITIES

Knowledge of the pulmonary system and the mechanisms and causes of pulmonary disease helps Federal agencies create effective regulations. Federal research in these areas is conducted mainly under the direction of EPA, the Department of Health and Human Services (DHHS), and the Department of Energy (DOE). EPA's Health Effects Research Laboratory (HERL) conducts research in pulmonary toxicology and epidemiology. DHHS conducts noncancer pulmonary research through several agencies, including the National Institutes of Health (NIH), the Centers for Disease Control (CDC), and the FDA. The Office of Health and Environmental Research, part of the Office of Energy Research, handles DOE's research in pulmonary toxicology.

Environmental Protection Agency

Two divisions within HERL conduct research on pulmonary toxicants. The Environmental Toxicology Division, through its Pulmonary Toxicology Branch, primarily tests the effects of air pollutants on animals to develop a basis for regulations under the CAA. In addition, it conducts pulmonary research with volatile organic compounds, sulfuric acid, and nitric acid. The Clinical Research Branch of the Human Studies Division conducts research on the effects on humans from exposures to ozone and other criteria pollutants regulated under CAA. The Epidemiology Branch of the Human Studies Division also carries out epidemiologic studies on the criteria pollutants.

HERL, located in Research Triangle Park, NC, collaborates with the University of North Carolina Center for Environmental Medicine and Lung Biology (CEMLB), which provides important support for the clinical and epidemiologic studies. HERL also works with the Duke University Center for Extrapolation Modeling, which works to confirm that animal models used in the Toxicology Division accurately predict responses in humans, and develops generic models to be used in risk assessment programs.

HERL's work in pulmonary toxicology takes several forms. The laboratory studies extrapolation techniques—applying knowledge gained from animal test results to human risk. HERL also performs acute exposure studies and attempts to apply those results to chronic exposure scenarios. HERL is engaged in the effort to define adversity of response, i.e., deciding at what point a response, which may be a normal compensatory activity of the body, can be considered "adverse." HERL also focuses on susceptible populations, such as asthmatics, to determine why some persons exhibit more detrimental effects from air pollution than others.

Current funding for the Pulmonary Toxicology Branch is approximately $2.6 million. The Clinical Research Branch is funded at a level of about $4.1 million, and the Epidemiology Branch receives approximately $2 .4 million (4,15).

Department of Health and Human Services

The National Institute of Environmental Health Sciences (NIEHS), part of the NIH, had a budget of approximately $5,230,000 for intramural noncancer pulmonary research in fiscal year 1991. NIEHS also made over $15 million in extamural grants to various universities and institutions in fiscal year 1991 for study of pulmonary toxicants. An additional $3,190,000 was spent on extramural contracts. The studies funded employ a wide range of techniques, including microbiology, whole animal studies, human clinical studies, and epidemiology. Substances researched include those affecting small sub-groups of the population, as well as those affecting the general population. The following projects provide examples of the extramural research funded by NIEHS.

- Scientists at the University of Iowa Department of Medicine received approximately $77,000 to study the effects of silica on the epithelial cells of the lungs in order to better understand how silicosis can be prevented.
- Researchers at the Medical College of Wisconsin received over $77,000 to study growth factor secretion in dust-induced lung disease in rats. This study was undertaken in order to clarify how alveolar

macrophages react to dust, eventually leading to pneumonconiosis.

- The National Jewish Center for Immunology and Respiratory Medicine received nearly $76,000 to study the immunologic and toxic mechanisms of beryllium disease in mice and humans in order to better understand the pathology of chronic beryllium disease in humans.
- Scientists at the University of California at Davis received $530,000 to study the effects of ozone on the lungs of rats, mice, hamsters, and monkeys as a basis to predict the effects of ozone in ambient air on humans.
- Researchers at the University of Rochester School of Medicine received $175,000 to conduct clinical inhalation studies on healthy humans and those with chronic pulmonary disease to investigate the respiratory effects of particulate and oxidant air pollutants (26).
- Scientists at the University of Iowa Pulmonary Disease Division received close to $53,000 to conduct epidemiologic studies of vegetable dust-induced airway disease in humans. The purpose of this study is to evaluate the feasibility of using the current threshold safety limit in the handling of cereal grain (oats, wheat, rye and barley) to protect the health of noncereal grain and vegetable (corn and soybean) handlers.
- Harvard University received $864,000 to conduct an epidemiologic study of the effects of acid aerosols, ozone, and particulate matter on the respiratory health of children in 24 cities in North America.

Using a model of asbestosis in laboratory animals, NIEHS intramural scientists have found that as macrophages engulf asbestos particles, growth factors are secreted that induce an increase in the number of fibroblasts. The fibrotic condition that results disrupts gas exchange. Current studies focus on stopping the release of the growth factors or preventing their biological activity. In fiscal year 1991, this project received funding of nearly $821,000 (19).

Other NIEHS intramural scientists are studying the regulation of the pulmonary surfactant system and its modification by toxic agents such as silica dusts. These studies are focused on identifying cellular factors released by inflammatory cells in response to a toxic agent that regulates surfactant production in alveolar Type II cells. This project received almost $575,000 in fiscal year 1991 (19).

NIEHS also contracts for a variety of inhalation toxicology studies on drugs, naturally occurring agents, and industrial compounds. For example, the IIT Research Institute in Chicago, IL, was awarded over $495,000 to investigate the toxicity of isobutyl nitrite (IBN). IBN is a component of some room deodorizers and is sold illicitly in ampules known as "Poppers." In the prechronic study, the lungs, bone-marrow, spleen, and nasal-cavity were identified as target organs for toxicity (19).

The National Heart, Lung, and Blood Institute (NHLBI), also part of NIH, conducts noncancer pulmonary research through its Division of Lung Diseases. This program includes studies on environmental lung disease caused by air pollutants and occupational lung disease. Approximately half of this research is carried out on animals and the other half is done on human subjects.

Extramural grants from NHLBI support research on pulmonary toxicology at a number of universities. Examples of environmental research include:

- Researchers at Louisiana State University are currently studying the effects of ozone, automobile exhaust, and tobacco smoke on the lung. This project is funded at approximately $127,000 per year.
- Scientists at the State University of New York at Stony Brook are studying ozone and respiratory mucus permeability, and receive about $79,000 for this project.
- Researchers at Pennsylvania State University are conducting tests on oxidant stress in the respiratory system at a funding level of approximately $185,000 per year.
- Two groups of scientists at the University of California at Irvine are conducting human research on inhaled particle deposition and animal research on the effects of air pollution. They receive approximately $325,000 per year for these studies.
- Researchers at the University of Maryland received approximately $100,000 to study the effect of environmental tobacco smoke on human lungs.
- Scientists at the University of California at Berkeley receive approximately $240,000 to conduct a human study of the physical and chemical proper-

ties of smoke and of the deposition of smoke particles in the lung.

- Researchers at Harvard University are conducting human and animal studies of inhaled retention of particulate matter, for which they receive approximately $134,000 per year.
- Scientists at the University of California at Santa Barbara received funding of about $190,000 for a study of the mechanisms of human response to ozone.

A number of research projects supported by NHLBI relate to occupational exposure to pulmonary toxicants. For example:

- Specialized Centers of Research (SCOR) investigators at the University of Iowa are studying the epidemiology and pulmonary responses to organic dust exposures in farm workers, for which they have received $127,000.
- The Iowa investigators and investigators at the University of New Mexico, are studying mechanisms of hypersensitivity pneumonitis, also known as farmer's lung, for which they have received over $135,000.
- A group of SCOR researchers at Tulane University received approximately $933,000 for a study of the respiratory effects of exposure to irritant gases and vapors in a population of 25,000 workers in the chemical manufacturing industry.
- At the University of Vermont, SCOR scientists received over $230,000 for an assessment of the mechanisms involved in injury and inflammation in occupationally related fibrotic lung disease associated with exposure to asbestos.
- Researchers at the State University of New York at Buffalo received $354,054 for a study of the pathogenesis of disease associated with exposures in the textile industry.

For fiscal years 1992 and 1993, the Division of Lung Diseases is developing two special initiatives. One is related to the mechanisms of ozone-induced lung injury and a second is on basic mechanisms of asbestos and nonasbestos fiber-related lung disease (13,14). NHLBI conducts basic research not specifically linked to any particular legislation or regulations. For fiscal year 1991, the total budget for lung research was $205,255,000; of that, $26,980,000 was dedicated to research on asthma, and approximately $22,619,000 was used to study chronic bronchitis and emphysema (12).

The National Institute for Occupational Safety and Health (NIOSH), part of the CDC, studies the pulmonary system through its Division of Respiratory Disease Studies (DRDS) at the Appalachian Laboratories for Occupational Health and Safety at Morgantown, WV. In addition, an extramural grant program is directed through NIOSH's administrative offices in Atlanta, GA. The overall budget for NIOSH in fiscal year 1992 is $103,450,000 with $13,400,000 designated for the study of occupational respiratory diseases. This is an increase from the approximately $7,687,112 allocated to intramural research and $3,196,218 spent on extramural research in the area of occupational lung disease in fiscal year 1991 (7,16).

NIOSH conducts research stimulated by the advice of DOL and investigator initiated research. Additionally, the Mine Health Research Advisory Committee suggests areas of study where gaps exist in the knowledge base. Other research suggestions come from NIOSH's Board of Scientific Counselors. NIOSH has specific authority from the OSH Act and FMSHA to conduct research and to make recommendations for health and safety standard regulations (27).

DRDS conducts epidemiologic research on pulmonary diseases related to the mining, milling, agricultural, construction, and other industries. Among the research programs in this area are a medical surveillance program for living coal miners (the National Coal Worker's X-ray Surveillance Program), and an autopsy program (the National Coal Workers' Autopsy Study) required by FMSHA. An ongoing surveillance program examines whether current coal mine dust standards protect miners' health. This study has continued for more than 20 years and is conducted through voluntary x-rays and an organized epidemiologic investigation. DRDS also conducts epidemiologic studies of occupational asthma and pulmonary disease caused by exposure to cotton dust. The agency monitors trends in the incidence of all occupational lung diseases. Clinical studies are conducted to determine the effects of occupational exposure to specific substances and to better understand human response mechanisms (28).

DRDS also conducts research in such areas as physiology, pathology, and microbiology to better understand the dangers of substances and the mechanisms of disease. Scientists choose animal models suitable for the study of particular agents and develop new laboratory techniques.

Extramural research is conducted through such programs as the NIOSH Centers for Agricultural Research, Education, and Disease and Injury Prevention Program. This program funds centers at the University of California at Davis, the University of Iowa at Iowa City, the National Farm Medicine Center in Marshfield, WI, and the Colorado State University at Fort Collins. Most of the program's pulmonary studies are conducted at the University of Iowa center, which conducts research in such areas as grain dust exposures and respiratory diseases in dairy farmers (7).

Unlike other Federal research agencies, NIOSH responds to requests from workers and their representatives to investigate the causes of accidents and illnesses in the workplace. In fiscal year 1992, NIOSH issued 40 final reports of respiratory disease health hazard evaluations. Onsite evaluations of possible pulmonary health hazards are performed by DRDS. DRDS medical personnel, industrial hygienists, and epidemiologists analyze the workplace situation and present suggestions for diminishing harmful exposures (28).

The National Center for Toxicological Research (NCTR) in Jefferson, AR, conducts methods development and toxicological research for the FDA. The purposes of the Center are to increase knowledge of human health risks associated with exposure to artificial and natural substances and to elucidate the mechanisms and impact of these risks. Pulmonary toxicity studies conducted at NCTR deal primarily with chronic long-term exposure to carcinogenic or mutagenic compounds. Currently research is focused on compounds of interest to FDA unrelated to pulmonary toxicity (1).

Department of Energy

DOE funds research on pulmonary toxicants conducted by the Inhalation Toxicology Research Institute (ITRI) in Albuquerque, NM. ITRI is owned by DOE and is operated under a long-term contract by a private,

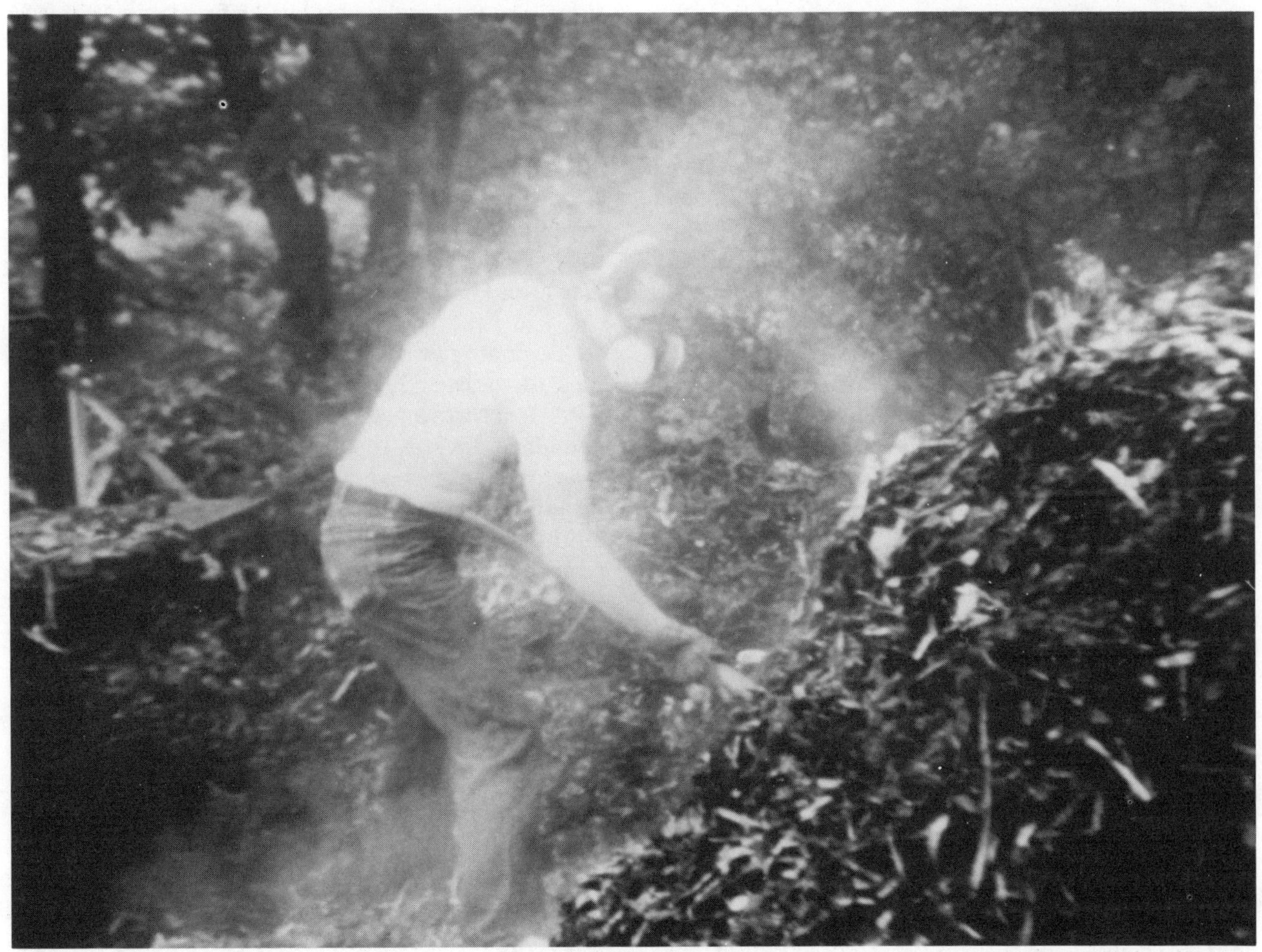

Photo Credit: G. Wagner, National Institute for Occupational Safety and Health

nonprofit corporate entity, the Lovelace Biomedical and Environmental Research Institute. ITRI receives approximately 75 percent of its funding from DOE, with the other 25 percent coming from other government agencies, nongovernment associations, and individual companies. Funding by DOE remains constant, while other government agencies and private sources provide funding for particular studies in areas of their interest.

All research at ITRI is lung related, and it ranges from molecular studies focusing on cellular changes caused by inhaled materials to clinical studies of human subjects. Studies are related to two general areas: those which examine the effects of specific substances on the respiratory system and those which explore the structure and function of the respiratory tract and the general behavior of gases, vapors, and particles in the respiratory tract (17).

Research on noncancer pulmonary toxicity is currently being conducted on ozone, nitrogen oxides, sulfur oxides, and the components of engine exhaust. Some studies focus on occupational exposures to pulmonary toxicants, including benzene, butadiene, nickel, and beryllium. Other research examines the effects of exposure to natural fibers, such as asbestos, and synthetic fibers, such as fiberglass. Studies on respiratory system structure and function focus on the uptake, deposition, and excretion of toxicants, and natural defenses of the respiratory system to inhaled materials (17).

ITRI proposes studies it decides need to be conducted, and DOE allocates funds according to its interests and resources. The scientific research budget for ITRI in fiscal year 1992 is approximately $13.5 million. In 1992 ITRI has allocated approximately 54 percent of its budget to cancer research. The other 46 percent is designated for noncancer research. Of the noncancer budget, a little over half is spent on general toxicology, including the study of the mechanisms of diseases, mathematical models of effects, and studies of the metabolism of compounds. Approximately one quarter of the budget is allocated for the study of the nature of airborne materials (vapors, particulate matter and gases). The remaining quarter is designated for dosimetry studies (18).

Cooperative Federal and Private Research

The Health Effects Institute (HEI) supports and evaluates research on the health effects of motor vehicle emissions. Its research program focuses on substances regulated by the NAAQS in the CAA, as well as other pollutants, such as diesel exhaust particles, methanol, and aldehydes (10). Because all research targets emissions, the majority of HEI's research focuses on the lung (20). All research at HEI is extramural, with funding mainly going to universities, but also to research centers (e.g., ITRI and the Los Amigos Research and Education Institute). Both cancer and noncancer research is funded, but no clear breakdown is available because research is pollutant-focused rather than effect-focused (29).

HEI receives one-half of its funding from EPA and the other half from all companies who make or sell automobiles, trucks, or engines in the United States. Currently, EPA and 28 private companies fund HEI. HEI bills the companies separately based proportionally on the number of vehicles or engines they sell that year in the United States. Contributing companies include American, European, and Japanese corporations. The total budget for HEI in fiscal year 1992 is $6 million (9).

A separate nonprofit organization, the Health Effects Research Institute—Asbestos Research (HEI-AR), was established in September 1989 to support scientific studies to evaluate airborne levels of asbestos in buildings, to assess exposure, and to examine asbestos handling and control strategies. HEI-AR is modeled after HEI but is an independent entity.

Beginning in fiscal year 1990 HEI-AR was scheduled to receive $2 million annually for 3 years from EPA. It secures an additional $2 million per year from combined sources in the real estate, insurance, and asbestos manufacturing industries, as well as from public and private organizations interested in asbestos. In 1991, HEI-AR published a report including a literature review of current knowledge of asbestos in buildings and identifying areas where more knowledge is needed. It has also begun a program of support and evaluation for scientific asbestos studies (11).

SUMMARY

The Federal Government plays an active role in the protection of pulmonary health through regulations and research. Regulations promulgated under the CAA, RCRA, TSCA, FIFRA, CPSA, and FDCA are designed to protect pulmonary health in the general population. Regulations promulgated under the OSH Act and FMSHA are designed to safeguard workers and miners respectively from exposure to pulmonary toxicants within the scope of their employment. Federal regulations call for a variety of measures to control the risk of exposure to pulmonary toxicants, including setting exposure levels, banning certain materials which pose an unmanageable risk of pulmonary injury, and requiring safety devices and education in the workplace.

Federal research on pulmonary toxicants is conducted primarily under the auspices of EPA, DHHS, and DOE. Research by these organizations is conducted on an intramural basis and on an extramural basis through grants to universities and other research institutes. An effort has been made to combine public and private funding of pulmonary toxicology research in HEI. Federally funded research includes studies involving human and animal subjects that employ research techniques ranging from cellular studies to epidemiology. Applying the knowledge gained through these studies, Federal agencies have been able to design regulations which should more effectively reduce health risks to the pulmonary system.

CHAPTER 4 REFERENCES

1. Adams, L., Office of Legislative Affairs, Food and Drug Administration, Washington, DC, personal communication, February 1992.
2. Anderson, F., *Environmental Protection: Law and Policy* (Boston, MA: Little, Brown & Co., 1990).
3. Blodgett, J., *Hazardous Air Pollutants: Revising Section 112 of the Clean Air Act,* Environment and Natural Resources Policy Division, Congressional Research Service, Library of Congress (Washington, DC: Library of Congress, February 1991).
4. Costa, D., Pulmonary Toxicology Branch, Health Effects Research Laboratory, U.S. Environmental Protection Agency, Research Triangle Park, NC, personal communication, September 1991.
5. 52 *Federal Register* 16022 (May 1, 1987).
6. 52 *Federal Register* 46766 (Nov. 6, 1990).
7. Friedlander, J., Centers for Disease Control, Atlanta, GA, personal communication, February 1992.
8. Hazen, S., 33/50 Program, Environmental Protection Agency, Washington, DC, personal communication, August 1991.
9. Health Effects Institute, "Annual Report: 1990-1991," unpublished booklet, Cambridge, MA.
10. Health Effects Institute, "Requests for Applications: 1991 Research Agenda," unpublished booklet, Cambridge, MA, October 1991.
11. Health Effects Institute—Asbestos Research, "Requests for Applications," unpublished booklet, Cambridge, MA, October 1990.
12. Hymiller, J., Budget Office, National Heart, Lung, and Blood Institute, National Institutes of Health, Washington, DC, personal communication, February 1992.
13. Kalica, A., Airways Division, National Heart, Lung, and Blood Institute, National Institutes of Health, Washington, DC, personal communication, February 1992.
14. Kiley, J., Airways Division, National Heart, Lung, and Blood Institute, National Institutes of Health, Washington, DC, personal communication, February 1992.
15. Koren, H., Health Effects Research Laboratories, U.S. Environmental Protection Agency, Research Triangle Park, NC, personal communication, March 1992.
16. Landry, M., Financial Management Office, Centers for Disease Control, Atlanta, GA, personal communication, November 1991.
17. Mauderly, J., Inhalation Toxicology Research Institute, Albuquerque, NM, personal communication, September 1991.
18. Mauderly, J., Inhalation Toxicology Research Institute, Albuquerque, NM, personal communication, January 1992.
19. Phelps, J., National Institute of Environmental Health Sciences, Research Triangle Park, NC, personal communication, February 1992.
20. Sivak, A., Health Effects Institute, Cambridge, MA, personal communication, January 1992.
21. U.S. Congress, *United States' Code Congressional and Administrative News,* 91st Cong., 1st Sess. (St. Paul, MN: West Publishing Co., 1969), p. 2506.
22. U.S. Congress, *United States' Code Congressional and Administrative News,* 95th Cong., 1st Sess. (St. Paul, MN: West Publishing Co., 1977), pp. 1187-97, 3405.
23. U.S. Congress, *United States' Code Congressional and Administrative News,* 101st Cong., 2d Sess. (St. Paul, MN: West Publishing Co., 1990), pp. 3392-94, 3513, 3518, 3532-50.
24. U.S. Environmental Protection Agency, Office of Air and Radiation, "Early Reduction Program," unpublished memo, Washington, DC, May 1991.
25. U.S. Environmental Protection Agency, "EPA's 33/50 Program: A Progress Report," unpublished memo, Washington, DC, July 1991.

26. Utell, M., University of Rochester Medical Center, Rochester, NY, personal communication, December 1991.

27. Wagner, G., Division of Respiratory Disease Studies, National Institute for Occupational Safety and Health, Morgantown, WV, personal communication, September 1991.

28. Wagner, G., Division of Respiratory Disease Studies, National Institute for Occupational Safety and Health, Morgantown, WV, personal communication, January 1992.

29. Warren, J., Health Effects Institute, Cambridge, MA, personal communication, February 1992.

Appendix

Glossary of Terms and Acronyms

Glossary

Alveolus/i: An air sac of the lungs at the termination of the bronchioles.

Antigen: A substance that brings about an immune response when introduced into the body.

Asthma: A chronic respiratory disease accompanied by labored breathing, chest constriction, and coughing.

Biologically effective dose: The amount of a contaminant that interacts with cells and results in altered physiologic function.

Black lung disease: An occupational disease of coal workers resulting from deposition of coal dust in the lungs.

Bronchoalveolar lavage fluid: Fluid obtained from the bronchoalveolar region of the lungs by lavage.

Bronchoconstriction: Narrowing of a bronchus caused by constriction of bronchial smooth muscle.

Bronchus: One of the large conducting air passages of the lungs commencing at the bifurcation of the trachea and terminating in the bronchioles.

Byssinosis: An occupational respiratory disease of cotton, flax, soft-hemp, and sisal workers characterized by symptoms of chest tightness.

Chronic bronchitis: Chronic inflammation of bronchi resulting in cough, sputum production, and often progressive breathlessness.

Cilia: Long slender microscopic structures extending from a cell surface and capable of rhythmic motion.

Collagen: Family of fibrous proteins.

Criteria pollutants: Airborne substances that may cause or contribute to air pollution and may reasonably be anticipated to endanger public health or welfare.

Cytotoxicity: The quality of being deadly to cells.

Dosimetry: The estimation of the amount of a toxicant that reaches the target site following exposure.

Elastin: The protein base of connective tissues.

Emphysema: A condition of the lungs characterized by labored breathing and increased susceptibility to infection.

Endothelium: The layer of cells lining the blood vessels.

Epidemiology: The scientific study of the distribution and occurrence of human diseases and health conditions and their determinants.

Epithelium: The thin layer of cells lining the inside of the respiratory tract.

Extrinsic allergic alveolitis: Severe immune responses to inhaled plant and animal dusts.

Fibroblast: The main cell of connective tissue.

Fibrosis: The formation of fibrous tissue as a result of injury or inflammation.

Gas exchange: The process of delivering oxygen in inhaled air to the bloodstream and delivering carbon dioxide and other gaseous components and metabolites in the blood stream to the exhalable air.

In vitro: Literally, in glass; pertaining to a biological process taking place in an artificial environment, usually a laboratory.

In vivo: Literally, in the living; pertaining to a biological process or reaction taking place in a living organism.

Larynx: Part of the respiratory tract containing the vocal cords.

Lavage: Irrigation or washing out of a cavity.

Macrophage: A type of large, amoeba-like cell, found in the blood and lymph, which ingests dead tissue, tumor cells, and foreign particles.

Magnetopneumography (MPG): A non-invasive technique which provides a means of actively monitoring the dust retained in the lungs of people exposed to magnetic or magnetizable dusts.

Microscopy: The use of an instrument to obtain magnified images of small objects.

Morphometry: The measurement of the structure and forms of organisms, as opposed to the measurement of their functions.

Mucus: The viscous fluid secreted by the mucous glands.

Nasopharyngeal region: Region of the lung comprising the nasal cavity and pharynx.

Phagocytosis: Consumption of foreign particles by cells.

Pharynx: The portion of the alimentary canal which intervenes between the mouth cavity and the esophagus and serves both for the passage of food and the performance of respiratory functions.

Pleura: The serous membrane lining the pulmonary cavity.

Pleural cavity: The space that separates the lungs from the chest wall. It contains a small amount of fluid and is bounded by membranes called the pleura.

Pneumoconiosis: A condition characterized by the deposition of mineral dust in the lungs as a result of occupational or environmental exposure.

Pulmonary edema: The accumulation of abnormally large amounts of watery fluid within the pulmonary alveoli.

Pulmonary fibrosis: The accumulation of abnormal quantities of fibrous tissue in the lung.

Pulmonary region: The region of the lung where oxygen in the air is supplied to the blood and carbon dioxide and other gaseous components and metabolites are released from the blood to the air remaining in the lungs.

Respiratory system: An interconnected series of air passages, cavernous organs, and cells that permit the introduction of oxygen, the exchange of gases, and the removal of carbon dioxide from the body as well as the production of speech.

Risk assessment: The analytical process by which the nature and magnitude of risk are identified. Four steps make up a complete risk assessment: hazard identification, dose-response assessment, exposure assessment, and risk characterization.

Secretory cells: Cells that secret mucus.

Spirometry: The measurement of the air inhaled and exhaled during respiration.

Toxicology: The study of adverse effects of natural or synthetic chemicals on living organisms.

Trachea: The windpipe.

Tracheobronchial region: The region of the lung comprising the trachea and bronchi.

Type I cells: Cells lining the alveoli which are very thin and delicate and spread over a relatively large area.

Type II cells: Cells lining the alveoli which release proteins and lipids providing a thin, fluid lining for the inside of the alveoli.

Acronyms

ATS	—American Thoracic Society
BAL	—Bronchoalveolar lavage
BALF	—Bronchoalveolar lavage fluid
CAA	—Clean Air Act
CASAC	—Clean Air Science Advisory Committee (EPA)
CDC	—Centers for Disease Control
CFR	—Code of Federal Regulations
CO	—Carbon monoxide
CO$_2$	—Carbon dioxide
COAD	—Chronic obstructive airway disease
COLD	—Chronic obstructive lung disease
COPD	—Chronic obstructive pulmonary disease
CPSA	—Consumer Product Safety Act
CPSC	—Consumer Product Safety Commission
DHHS	—Department of Health and Human Services
DL$_{CO}$	—Diffusing capacity of the lung for carbon monoxide
DOE	—Department of Energy
DRDS	—Division of Respiratory Disease Studies (NIOSH)
EPA	—Environmental Protection Agency
ERP	—Early Reduction Program
FDA	—Food and Drug Administration
FDCA	—Food, Drug, and Cosmetic Act
FEF$_{50}$	—Forced expiratory flow of 50 percent
FEF$_{75}$	—Forced expiratory flow of 75 percent
FEV$_1$	—Forced expiratory volume in 1 second
FHSA	—Federal Hazardous Substances Act
FIFRA	—Federal Insecticide, Fungicide, and Rodenticide Act
FMSHA	—Federal Mine Safety and Health Act
FVC	—Forced vital capacity
HEI	—Health Effects Institute
HERL	—Health Effects Research Laboratory
ITRI	—Inhalation Toxicology Research Institute
MACT	—Maximum achievable control technology
MMEF	—Maximal midexpiratory flow
MPG	—Magnetopneumography
MSHA	—Mine Safety and Health Administration
NAAQS	—National Ambient Air Quality Standards
NAS	—National Academy of Sciences
NCTR	—National Center for Toxicological Research
NHLBI	—National Heart, Lung, and Blood Institute
NIEHS	—National Institute of Environmental Health Sciences
NIH	—National Institutes of Health
NIOSH	—National Institute for Occupational Safety and Health
NO$_x$	—Nitrogen oxides
NRC	—National Research Council
OSHA	—Occupational Safety and Health Administration
OTA	—Office of Technology Assessment
PEL	—Permissible exposure limit
RCRA	—Resource Conservation and Recovery Act
TRI	—Toxics Release Inventory
TSCA	—Toxic Substances Control Act
UCLA	—University of California at Los Angeles
VOC	—Volatile organic compounds

Index

U.S. GOVERNMENT PRINTING OFFICE : 1992 O - 297-932 : QL 3

Superintendent of Documents **Publications** Order Form

Order Processing Code:
* **6281**

☐ **YES**, please send me the following:

Charge your order.
It's Easy!

To fax your orders (202) 512–2250

P3

__________ copies of *Identifying and Controlling Pulmonary Toxicants (88 pages)*
S/N 052-003-01285-5 at $4.25 each.

The total cost of my order is $__________. International customers please add 25%. Prices include regular domestic postage and handling and are subject to change.

____
(Company or Personal Name)   (Please type or print)

____
(Additional address/attention line)

____
(Street address)

____
(City, State, ZIP Code)

____
(Daytime phone including area code)

____
(Purchase Order No.)

May we make your name/address available to other mailers? YES ☐ NO ☐

Please Choose Method of Payment:

☐ Check Payable to the Superintendent of Documents

☐ GPO Deposit Account ☐☐☐☐☐☐☐ – ☐

☐ VISA or MasterCard Account

☐☐☐☐☐☐☐☐☐☐☐☐☐☐☐☐☐☐☐☐

☐☐☐☐ (Credit card expiration date)

Thank you for your order!

____
(Authorizing Signature)   6/92

Mail To: New Orders, Superintendent of Documents
P.O. Box 371954, Pittsburgh, PA 15250–7954